$2.
LT

LYN REVSON'S WORLD OF STYLE

LYN REVSON'S WORLD OF STYLE

How to Join It and Live It

by Lyn Revson

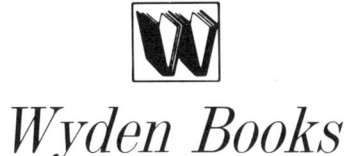

Wyden Books

Copyright © 1977 by Lyn Revson

All rights reserved. No part of this book may be reproduced, stored in a retrieval system or transmitted in any form by an electronic, mechanical, photocopying, recording means or otherwise, without prior written permission of the author. Manufactured in the United States of America.

FIRST EDITION

*Trade distribution by Simon and Schuster
A Division of Gulf + Western Corporation
New York, New York 10020*

Designed by Tere LoPrete

Library of Congress Cataloging in Publication Data

Revson, Lyn.
    Lyn Revson's world of style.
    1. Fashion.   2. Beauty, Personal.   3. Entertaining.   4. Women—Conduct of life.
I. Title.
TT.507.R47   646.7   77-14945
ISBN 0-671-22954-0

FOR MY CHILDREN
Steven, Jeffrey, and Susan

Contents

1	*How It All Begins—and Ends*	3
2	*Looking Your Best*	5
	"Working" at Your Look—How Hard and How Much?	6
	My Personal "Beauty Routine"	7
	Eating for Beauty	13
	Keeping Your Weight Where It Belongs	13
	How to Stay Thin Without Going on a Diet	14
	How Thin Is Too Thin?	16
	The Beauty-Making Benefits of Exercise	17
	Sleep, Beautiful Sleep	20
	Smoking and Drinking and Why They're Bad for Your Looks	20
	Upper and Downer People	22
	Makeup: Finding What's Best for You	25
	A Few Basic Makeup Dos and Don'ts	28
	Your Hair and How to Find the Best Way to Wear It	30
	How to Choose a Hairstyle	36
	How to Care for Your Hair	38

How to Choose a Good Hairdresser	40
A Few Words about Teeth	42
Fragrance: How to Choose It and Wear It	46
How to Stop Worrying about Your Looks—and Why	50

3 Dressing Well 52

Style vs. Fashion	54
Dress to Please Yourself	57
How to Have "Clothes Sense"	59
Fashion Mistakes and How to Learn from Them	69
How to Build a Wardrobe	72
A Few Dos and Don'ts for Building a Wardrobe	81
How to Shop Wisely and Well	83
What to Wear Where	90
A Few Fashions to Avoid	101
A Final Word about Money and Clothes	104

4 Friends and Other People 106

How to Cultivate People for Fun and Profit	107
Invitations: When to Say Yes, When to Say No, and How to Say Either	111
How to Go Out "As Well as You Can"	113
How to Know if You're a Bore and What to Do About It	121
How to Deal with a Bore	123
What to Do about a Boring Friend	124
When You Go as a Couple	126
How to Handle the Marijuana Question	128
The Evening that Never Gets Off the Ground	128
How and When to Leave	130
Special Gifts for Special People	131
How Not to Get Caught in the Christmas Crush	140
Wrappings That Say You	140

	What to Buy for the Person Who "Has Everything"	141
	A Few Thoughts about Gifts and Children	143
	Getting Your Message Across: Phone Calls, Notes, and Letters	145
5	***Managing***	***148***
	First Things First	149
	How to Plan a No-Fail (or Almost) Party Guest List	150
	Party Food: Serving with Style	152
	Organizing for a Party—Step by Step by Step	156
	Children at the Table?	162
	The Helpers in Your Life and How to Work with Them	162
	Quick Getaways: How to Pack like a Pro	166
	House Guesting: Your Place and Theirs	170
	The All-Important Decorator	172
	Charity Begins at . . .	177
6	***My Favorite People, Places, and Things***	***183***
	Motherhood	183
	Places and Things	185
	Venice	185
	Israel	188
	Palm Springs	190
	Paris, London, Rome	191
	New York	193
	New York Restaurants	193
	The Tall Ships	195
	Cooking	195
	Houston	197
	Cape Kennedy and the Apollo 13 Launch	198
	Atlantic City	199
	Disneyland	199

Superbowl	199
Montreal	200
Barbados	202
Jones Beach	202
Marriage	205

LYN REVSON'S
WORLD OF STYLE

1
How It All Begins—and Ends

They tell me I have style. I've heard and read that now so often that I'm beginning to think there must be some truth to the rumor.

Certainly I think that I have my own very personal Lyn way of running my life, and I know that my way works for me and the people I value. There's nothing complicated or mysterious about my way, because I'm not a complicated or mysterious person. In all areas of my life—in fashion, beauty, entertaining, traveling, running a home, and just about everything else—I always tried to find the simplest, best, most direct way of getting things done.

Most things involve choices, and all of them involve giving up something. I find my energy keeps leaking away when I'm in a state of indecision; therefore, I find it best not to live my life with "I should have," "could have," etc. Once I make a decision, I function best when I don't look to the left or right of me, or question my choice.

If that's my style, and I suppose it is, then that's what this book is all about: using your head and making the most of what you have, then melting and immersing yourself in the present situation and enjoying and learning from it.

It's worked well for me and I pass it along to you.

2

Looking Your Best

Some women make a "career" out of beauty. Their days are planned around hair appointments and facials, manicures, visits to an exercise class, visits from their personal masseuse. You can always spot the "career beauty" by her curiously blank expression: she hardly ever frowns or even laughs because she's afraid of putting lines on her face. Another dead giveaway is the ultra-careful way she has of switching on a light, dialing a telephone, zipping a zipper. One of her great fears is to break a fingernail.

The women I have in mind are not professional models or actresses. They're basically rather ordinary creatures with a certain amount of time and money on their hands—time and money which they've chosen to invest in making themselves look more beautiful.

There's nothing wrong with that goal. But the beautiful person who contributes only her physical presence (no matter how gorgeous) to a party, to the lives of the people she's close to, to the world at large, becomes just a decorative object. "A piece of Louis XIV furniture," as one of my friends puts it. Lovely, but just part of the background, never right there at the very center making things happen.

"Working" at Your Look—How Hard and How Much?

The woman with real style is never just a piece of furniture. She's a living, breathing, laughing, crying human being whose presence is always felt. Former *Vogue* editor Diana Vreeland is like that. A great beauty? Never! But a woman of enormous personal style, wit, and verve. When she walks into a room, you know she's there.

You can have great style without physical beauty. In fact, any woman who thinks all she has to do to achieve a certain style is to work on her looks is mistaken. The world is full of beautiful (or would-be beautiful) people with a style rating of zero. I come across them practically every day of my life.

Not that taking good care of yourself and your appearance isn't important. Looking good and feeling good are *very* important. Think about the women you know who have let themselves go, who never (or hardly ever) bother about their hair, their skin, or their figures. That kind of woman often says she's "too busy" to do anything about her looks; she's got other, more important things to do. Or maybe she says she simply doesn't care. (I have the feeling that most of these women worry that they'll be thought "shallow" if they show concern for their looks. Strange: it doesn't seem to bother them to be considered "sloppy.")

I may be wrong, but I believe women who say they don't care at all about their appearance are really very unhappy about themselves. Yet they're terrified of trying to change. If they don't try, they'll never fail. But they'll also never have the satisfaction of succeeding either. (This applies to everything, of course, and not just to improving one's looks.)

I don't know about you, but as a woman, I probably wouldn't seek out the "afraid to try" female as a friend. I doubt that many men are turned on by her either.

I suppose what it all comes down to is that in matters of beauty (as in just about everything else) a certain practical, realistic attitude is called for. Trying too hard, devoting all of your time and energy to the cause, can be self-defeating. It can turn you into a store window dummy or a "piece of furniture." But not trying at all is just as bad.

Just how hard *should* you work at your looks? That's a question nobody can answer for you in specific terms. I'm always amused when I read in a magazine or beauty book that *all* women should have a once-a-week facial. (I've *never* had a facial.) Or that hair *must* be trimmed every six weeks. (Once a year is more like it for me.) Or that *everyone* needs to wear a moisturizer under their makeup. (I'm lucky. My skin is oily, so I don't need a moisturizer.) We all have specific needs and priorities. The idea of telling women they *must* spend at least five minutes on this and ten minutes on that, or that they need to establish elaborate and rigid beauty routines, strikes me as presumptuous.

Talking this over frankly with some of the many busy and beautiful women I know, I've come to the conclusion that the ones who have the most going for them are not necessarily the ones who "work hard at their looks" and have complicated "beauty routines." Instead, they're the ones who've learned to make the most of what they have in the easiest, least-time-consuming ways.

Like them, if you're going to make the most of your looks, you're going to have to set aside *some* time each day to work at it. But how much or how little time depends on what kind of improvements you're trying to make, as well as on all the other big and little things that are going on in your life.

My Personal "Beauty Routine"

Would you like to know about my own personal beauty routine?

Well, I'm usually up and out of bed sometime between eight and nine o'clock in the morning. I don't walk over to a full-length mirror and say to myself, "Good morning and aren't you beautiful today," as one beauty-book writer suggests. (A suggestion, I assume, which is supposed to put you in a "beautiful" frame of mind for the remainder of the day.) First I feed my fish, then I open the shutters and look out of the window. Then I clean my teeth, run a brush through my hair, and wash my face with soap and a washcloth.

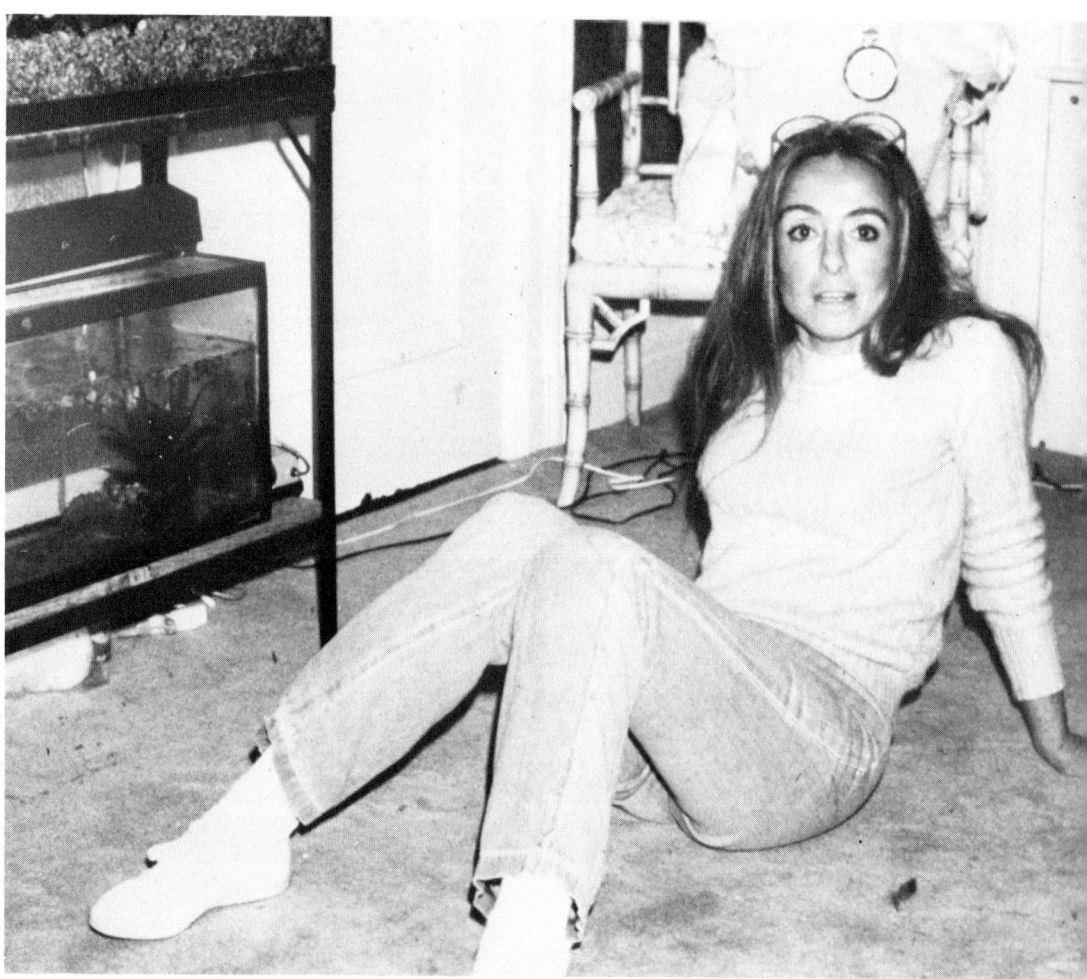

My "complicated beauty routine" starts with waking up in the morning and feeding my fish. (PHOTO: LEE GUBER)

Next I have breakfast, usually just juice and coffee, sometimes a bagel and cream cheese and bacon. Yes, I'm aware of what they say about breakfast. I know it's supposed to be the most important meal of the day. But the truth is, I'm not hungry first thing in the morning, and I'd rather eat more of what I like later on, when I'll enjoy it. (Also, I've never liked eggs—maybe because my mother always used to try and force them on me when I was little. Soft-boiled eggs with things that hung. Ugh!)

During breakfast, I read through as much of *The New York Times* and the *Wall Street Journal* as possible. Now there's a very important beauty tip for you: know what's happening in the world. Be informed. Take an interest. It may not give you a sexier smile or a more graceful figure, but it will help make you a more sparkling guest, hostess, date, or whatever.

If it's a busy day, I've got my clothes on and my makeup (more about that shortly) and I'm out of the house within half an hour. If I have more time, I do my exercises before leaving. They take about twenty minutes, and that's about as specific as I'll be about my exercises here—not because there's anything secret about them, but because they were especially prescribed for me to strengthen my back, which tends to be weak and gives me occasional pain.

(This isn't to say that I wouldn't exercise if I didn't have the back problem. I've exercised regularly for more than thirty years and I'm a firm believer in exercise for everyone. It helps you stay fit and trim. Just as important, it contributes to a feeling of well-being. Exercise is probably the most important part of anyone's beauty routine. The fact that I have a back problem only makes exercise all the more important to me; if I skip the exercise, even for a few days, I suffer.)

That's about it for the morning part of my "routine." If I'm going out at night, I try to lie down for twenty minutes or so before dressing for the evening. The idea of a short rest before going out makes wonderful sense. Lying down in a darkened room and turning your mind off, even if you don't actually fall asleep, is marvelously refreshing. I know I definitely look and feel better when I'm able to do it. The trouble is, I often don't have the time. And when I do have time, it's hard for me to stay still and really relax. I crawl into bed, close my eyes, and the next thing I know my mind is racing ahead to the following day's schedule. I try to force myself to lie still and rest by focusing on something lovely and peaceful, like a sandy beach on a sunny day. Finally, I look at the clock. If I'm lucky, I've "rested" for seven or eight minutes.

I do always bathe before going out at night. I don't use bubble bath or bath salts because their scent interferes with the fragrance I use. Also, though my complexion tends to be oily, the skin on the rest of my body is dry from too much sun and too many baths. I've found a wonderful skin treatment called Alpha Keri Bath Oil. It soothes and smooths my skin without making it feel greasy, and it's unscented, so it doesn't clash with my fragrance. When I get out of the tub, I rub in some Lubriderm Lotion, another unscented nongreasy product for dry skin. (My skin really *is* parched.)

After bathing, I do my makeup, dress, and spray on some Bal à Versailles, and I'm ready to go.

On evenings when I'm staying home alone, I simply bathe, get into my robe, and settle down with something to read. There are always five or six books that I'm anxious to get through, and these quiet evenings are, for me, a great treat. I rarely stay up late when I'm home alone, so at ten thirty or so, I brush my hair, clean my teeth, and hop into bed. And that, my friends, is Lyn Revson's mysterious, exotic beauty routine.

Of course I do other things. Once a week I go to Marc Sinclaire at Elizabeth Arden for a shampoo. I do as much walking as I can and I often spend Saturday or Sunday bicycling in Central Park. I ski in the winter and play tennis all year round and I've recently taken up running. (One of my greatest thrills this year was entering a four-mile race held in Central Park. Of 530 starters, 517 completed the race and—you guessed it—I was the 517th runner to cross the finish line. Now I'm working on my speed and endurance, and believe me, next year I won't be the last!)

The point is, I *don't* do anything complicated. In fact, I probably should work harder at my looks. I know I could treat my skin more kindly. (I love the look of a deep, dark tan; sometimes I even take a reflector with me to the beach and sneak off with it so that I can use

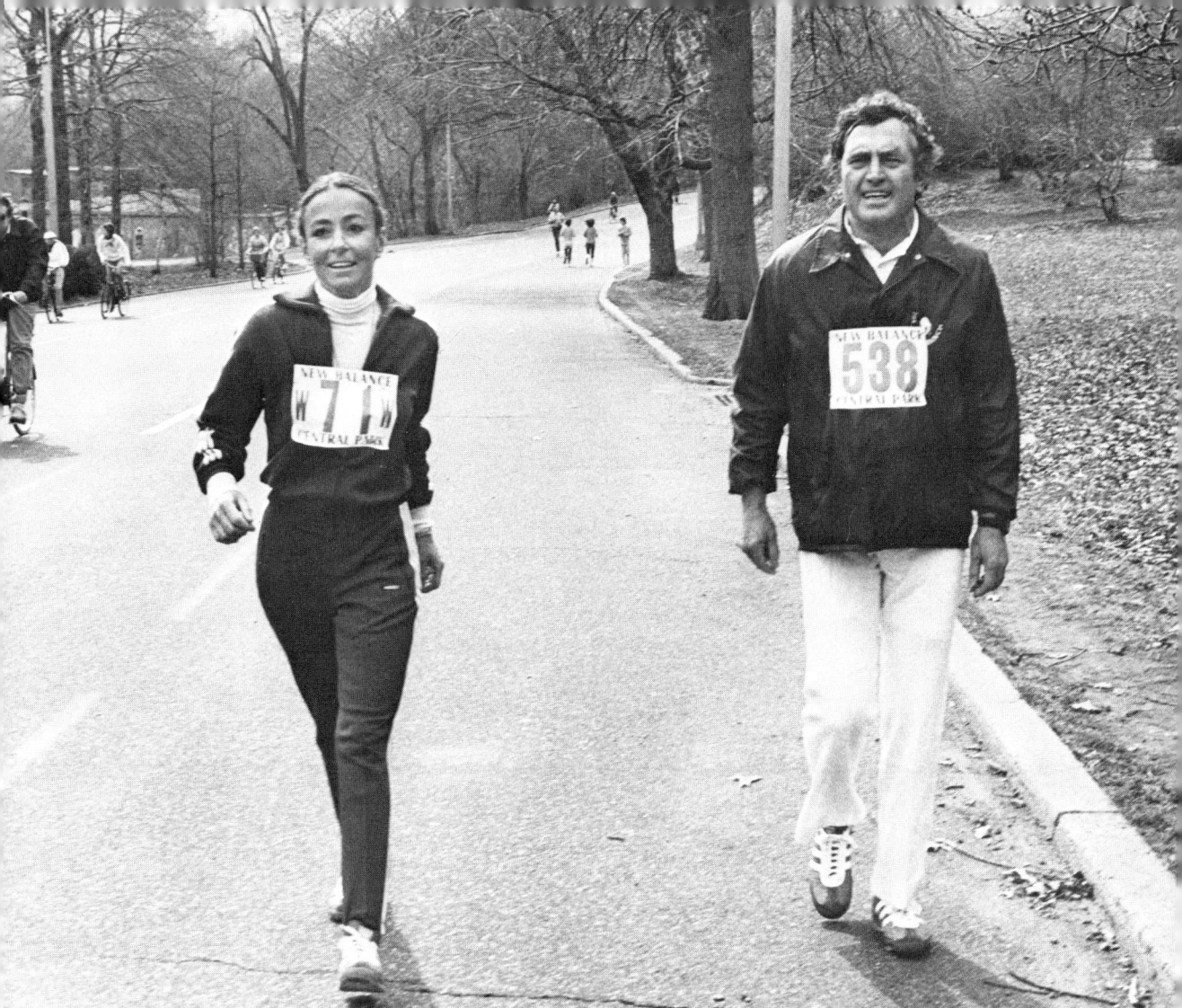

Running is marvelous exercise. Here, my friend Lee Guber cheers me on as I finish my first race. (PHOTO: SHARON SOPHER)

it without somebody catching me and giving me a lecture about the harmful effects of concentrating the sun's rays on the skin. But Marlon Brando knew, all right. Once at a charity party he walked up to me and said, "You're either an Indian or you use a reflector."

Perhaps the reason I'm able to get away with doing so little on a day-to-day basis is that I have very healthy habits in general. No, I'm not a health nut. I am, though, very fortunate in that I never had

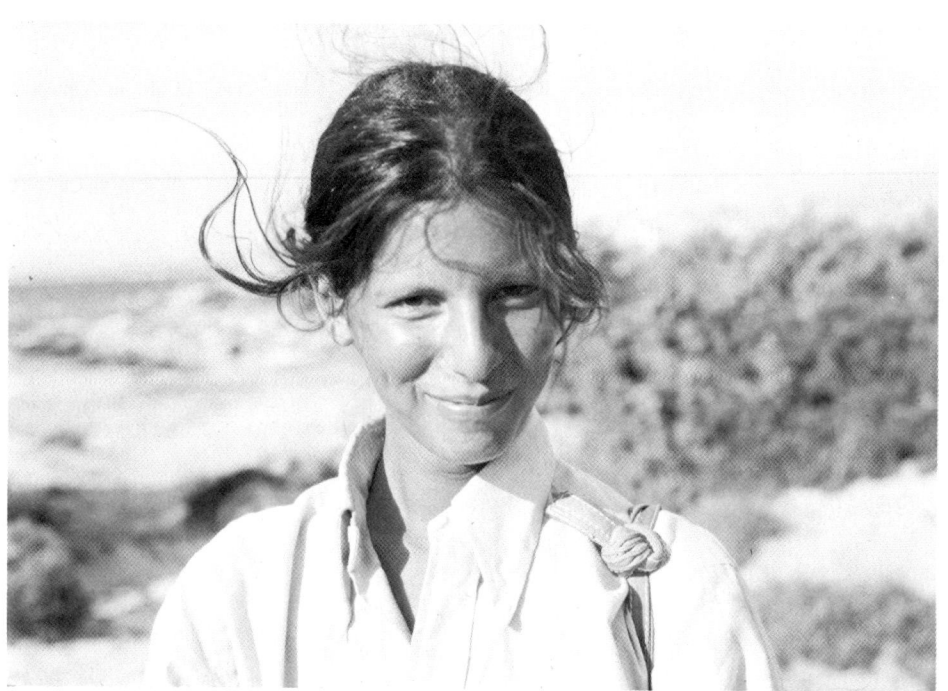

My daughter Susan, now 22, loves the sun as much as I do. Here she is in California, hair pinned up, no makeup; here I am in Atlantic City, hair pinned up, no makeup. Like mother, like daughter. (PHOTO: LEE GUBER)

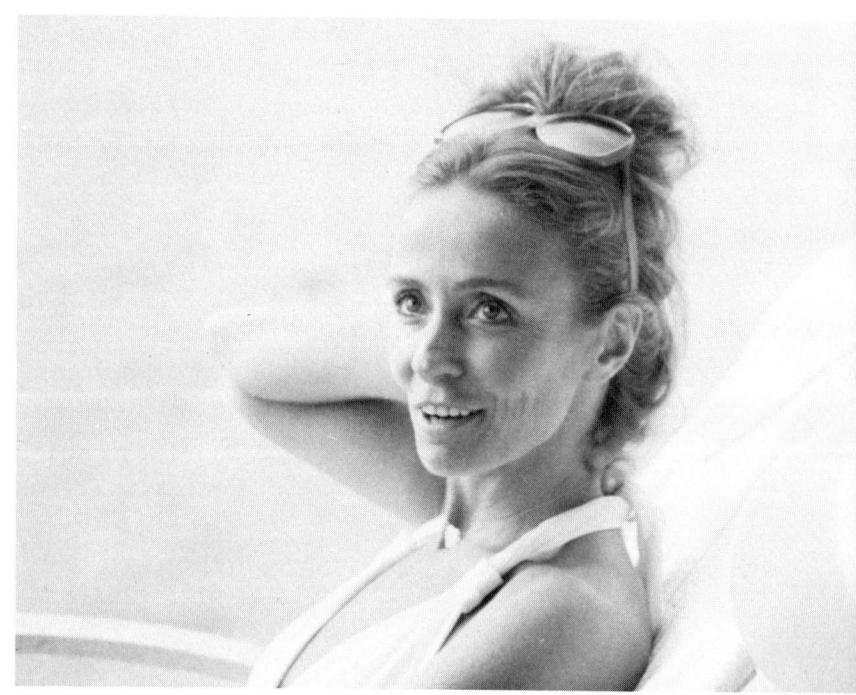

a strong urge to smoke or drink. In the long run, no beauty routine yet devised can make up for so-so health and fitness.

So, instead of giving out a lot of specific beauty tips, I'm going to start by suggesting a few ways to achieve better health and fitness.

Eating for Beauty

The woman who isn't getting enough of all the essential nutrients her body needs for good health can't possibly feel and look her best.

I've always been an "up" person with lots of energy, and in general, except for an occasional bout of laryngitis and my bad back and neck, my health has been excellent. (I've never been in a hospital except to have my children. I'm very lucky.) In any event, poor nutrition was never a problem. However, I do have friends who swear that a switch to more sensible eating habits helped put the bounce back into their step and healthy new life in their skin and hair.

I'm not an expert on nutrition and I wouldn't presume to tell anyone how to eat for maximum health and vitality. That's the kind of information that must come from your doctor. But if you're feeling sluggish and your hair doesn't shine and your skin looks dull and tired, by all means have a checkup. Assuming nothing is drastically wrong, it could be that your eating habits leave something to be desired. Perhaps your doctor can make a few suggestions for improving them—and your looks.

Keeping Your Weight Where It Belongs

We all know: styles in beauty change just as clothing styles do. Throughout history there have been "fat" cycles—times when the rounded, well-fleshed woman was the ideal—and "thin" cycles.

Today we're in a thin cycle. A slender figure is not only more pleasing to the modern eye, we also know now that it's healthier to be thin. Staying slender is more than just a matter of style.

There are plenty of good diets available to anyone who wants to lose weight. (A favorite with several women I know is the *Harper's Bazaar* Diet. Write to them and they'll send you a copy.)

There are also a lot of bad diets. How can you tell the good from the bad? Well, a good diet always includes a variety of different kinds of foods, which means that even though you consume fewer calories, your body continues to be supplied with enough of all the protein, vitamins, and minerals it needs for good health. The diets to avoid are the ones that feature just one or two different food groups (the all-protein diet, for example, or the all-carbohydrate diet). You may lose weight on one of these fad diets. But you might also end up with lackluster hair, a complexion that's lost its freshness and bloom, and a generally listless, rundown feeling because your body hasn't been getting all the things it needs to stay in top condition.

If you're planning to lose more than ten or fifteen pounds, the best advice anyone can give you is to suggest that you check with a good doctor and see what kind of diet he or she recommends. And for heaven's sake, be satisfied with a slow, steady weight loss. You may want desperately to be in bikini shape by summer, but do you also want the flabby, loose skin that so often accompanies a too-rapid weight loss? Think twice about it. And by all means exercise to help keep your body firm as you lose.

How to Stay Thin Without Going on a Diet

As for me, I hardly ever "go on a diet" in the usual sense. Over the years I've discovered a painless way to stay at or about my ideal weight. It only requires a bathroom scale and some periodic self-discipline. I'll explain:

At 5 feet 5 1/2 inches tall, I look and feel my best when I weigh between 116 and 118 pounds. First thing in the morning, every other day, I step on the scale. If the needle registers 118, 119, or even 120, fine, no problem. But when it gets up to 121 or 122, I know it's time to start watching myself, and I do. Usually I can coax the needle back down to 118 within a couple of days simply by getting more exercise and eating less in the way of pasta, bread, and candy. (Yes, I have to confess I love "junk food." There are jars of jelly beans and brown licorice in my bedroom and boxes of Milky Ways in the refrigerator. Is it any wonder my dentist is one of my best friends?)

I find it's not difficult to give up my favorite foods when I know it's only for a little while.

The trick is never to allow a small problem to grow into a large one. Two or three pounds are easy to deal with. Five pounds or more is something else again. I know. I spent some time a couple of summers ago blissfully neglectful of my weight-watching system. Lolling around on the beach all day in a bathing suit, wearing mostly jeans at night, eating lots of spaghetti, ice cream, pizza—well, when I got back to New York in September and tried on some of my city clothes, I discovered all my waistbands had "shrunk" by a good inch and a half. It was only a five-pound weight gain, but it took two months of

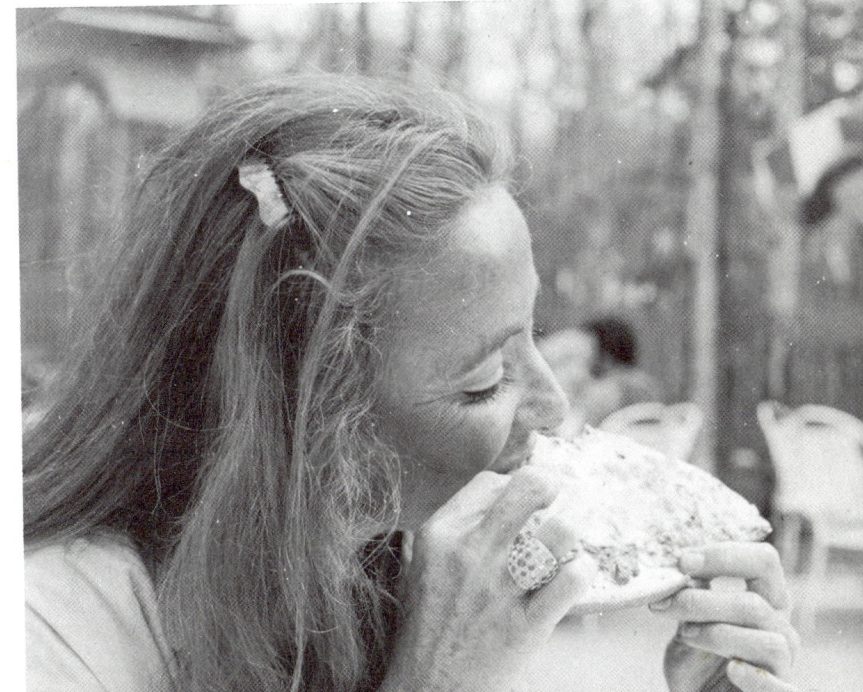

It's a good thing I exercise so much. With my appetite for pizza, I'd be in terrible shape if I didn't. (In some circles I'm known as the "pizza queen.") (PHOTO: LEE GUBER)

disciplined exercise and strict diet before my clothes fit comfortably. I will never allow that to happen again.

How Thin Is Too Thin?

To some women emaciation equals elegance. They're so obsessed with the idea of thinness, they diet themselves down to the point of being grotesque.

It's true, the thin woman looks younger and better in her clothes than the woman who weighs twenty pounds more than she should. But there's nothing attractive about a face that's gaunt and haggard from too much dieting, or knees and elbows that jut out like hooks to hang hats on. I've known women who've dieted down to practically nothing and were positively delighted with their starved "concentration camp" look. I always wonder what they see when they look at themselves in the mirror. It couldn't possibly be the same image that the rest of the world sees.

How thin you want to be is ultimately up to you, of course. But my suggestion is not to get too carried away with dieting, especially if you're of what they used to call "a certain age" (which could be anywhere from thirty on up). Losing too much weight will accentuate any little wrinkles and lines you already have on your face and helps speed up the formation of new ones. Let's also not forget how important breasts and hips are as female equipment. Even most top fashion models have a little something to sit down on. A few months ago, when I'd been playing a lot of tennis, burning off more calories than usual and not making up for it by eating more, a male friend took a good, long look at me and said, "Hey, where did you leave your ass?"

I know that some women diet past the point of attractiveness because they've got a thing about reducing certain parts of their bodies. The woman who has lost weight but whose breasts are still disproportionately large may hope that if she loses "just a few more pounds," she won't be top-heavy anymore. The woman with a relatively big behind or heavy thighs hopes the next few pounds will be shed from those areas of her anatomy. Usually, it doesn't work out that way. *Some* weight will be lost from the problem areas, but chances are the *proportions* will stay pretty much the same.

What do you do if you've dieted down to your ideal weight or a few pounds below and you're still stuck with breasts or thighs or hips that are out of proportion to the rest of your body? First, try exercises that are especially designed for spot reducing. (You'll find them in many of the dozens of exercise books on the market.) Give them a chance to work. It may take months for results to show up.

If exercise doesn't work, try to live with your less than ideal shape. (Remember, what looms in your mind as a major figure flaw may be hardly noticeable to others.) If that's impossible, if you absolutely can't accept your body as it is, investigate the possibility of plastic surgery. Surgical "figure molding" is expensive, uncomfortable, and risky; it should not be undertaken without a lot of thought. But if your body is a source of constant unhappiness and embarrassment, it may be worth your while at least to discuss your problem with a doctor qualified to do something about it.

The Beauty-Making Benefits of Exercise

You already know my feelings about exercise. It's essential for any woman who wants to look and feel her best. It firms and tones your muscles. It burns off extra calories. It revs up circulation. It makes you glow from head to toe. It also relieves tension. And afterward, there's that wonderful feeling of well-being. But here's another thing about exercise: far from draining your energy reserves, it seems to add to them. People who start on a regular exercise program are often amazed at how much *less* fatigued they are at the end of the day than before—how much *more* they enjoy going out, or having people over in the evening.

Doctors have known for years about the health and beauty-making benefits of exercise. But until quite recently, if you took your jogging, your cycling, or your tennis playing very seriously, you ran the risk of being thought of as a bit of an oddball. Now those very same activities are "very in." The same people who, a couple of years ago, said they'd love to exercise but didn't have the time for it, now *make* the time. I don't know what it's like where you live, but early every weekday morning in my neighborhood the sidewalks along Central Park thump with the sound of running shoes as lawyers, stockbrokers, theatrical producers, actresses, models, all in bright red, blue, or green sweat suits, do a lap or two before breakfast and dressing for work.

Of course, jogging and bicycling and tennis aren't the only ways to stay in shape. Walking is good and so are vigorous stretch-and-bend calisthenics. In fact, almost any brisk activity done on a regular basis can be a big health and beauty plus.

Incidentally, that word "regular" is important. Exercise won't do much good if it isn't done consistently, according to plan. If you're going to work out three times a week, stop for two weeks, take it up again once a week, and then skip it for a month, you may as well save yourself the trouble of all that heavy breathing. Whatever your routine—once a day, every other day, or three times a week—you have to adhere to it faithfully.

If you want to plan a fitness program suited to your needs and life-style (and I hope you do), there are dozens of books on the subject to help you get started. The ones I like the best are by Marjorie Craig, particularly *Miss Craig's Twenty-one Day Shape Up Program for Men and Women* (Random House, 1968). Almost all of these books caution the person who has been sitting around leading a basically sedentary life for years to go slowly at first. It's always a good idea to check with your doctor before embarking on any new program of physical activity.

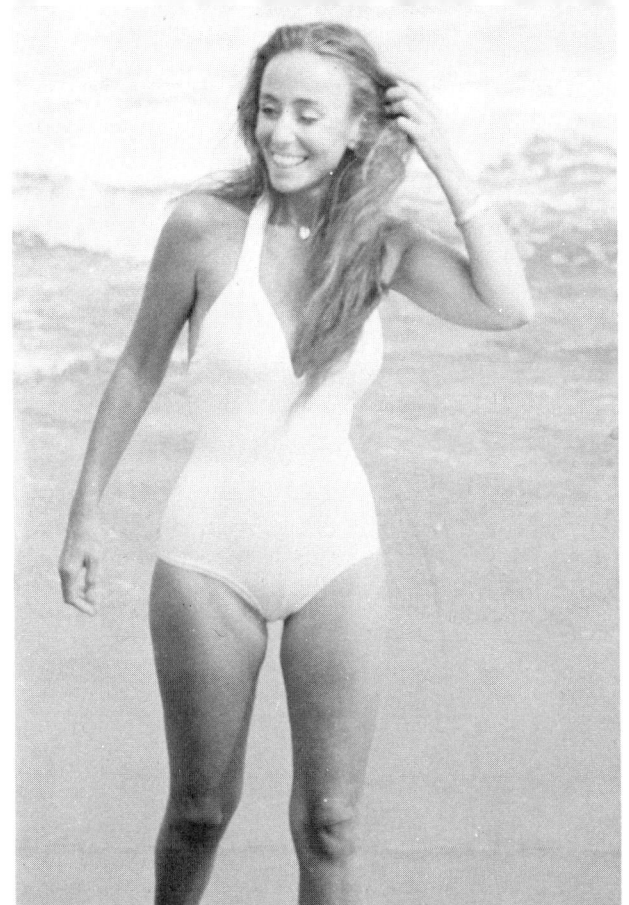

Looks like I just swam the English Channel, and I wish I had. Swimming is such wonderful exercise. But the truth is, I don't swim a stroke. (PHOTO: LEE GUBER)

Bicycling is another great way to exercise. On Saturday mornings when the weather is fine, I bike two or three times around Central Park... then collapse on the grass with a hot dog and grape soda. (PHOTO: LEE GUBER)

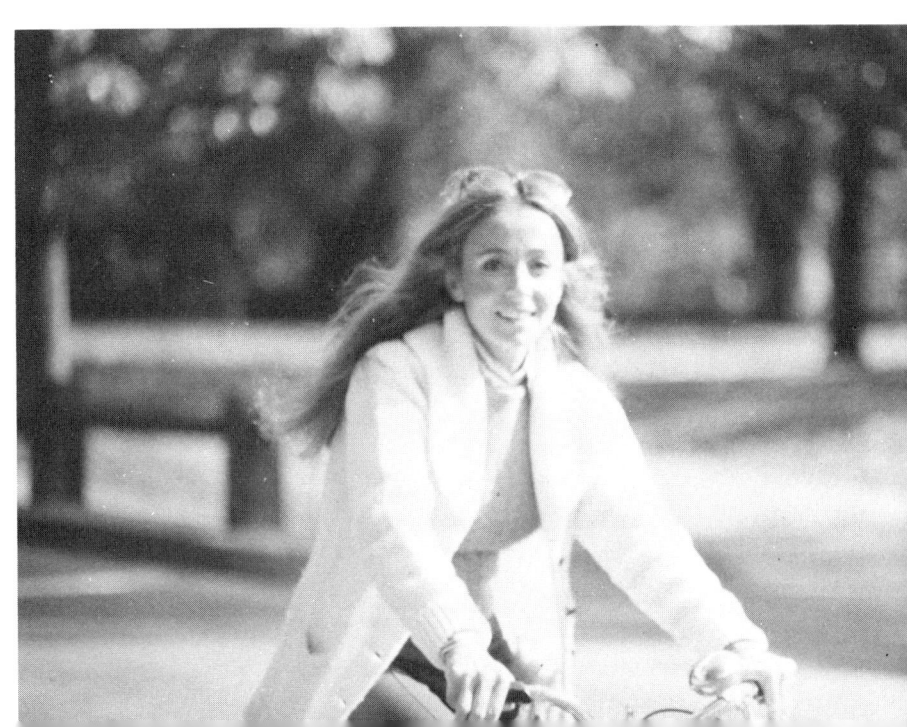

Sleep, Beautiful Sleep

If you can stay out till two every night without dragging around all the next day looking drawn and feeling exhausted, more power to you. I can't do it. I need my sleep. And since I'm not the napping type to begin with—most days I truly am too busy to lie down and rest anyway—I make sure I get enough sleep at night. It's the rare party that keeps me out past midnight on a weekday, and I don't mind being the first to leave. After all, someone has to leave first, and I've noticed that the person who has the good sense to know when the party is over and then makes the first move to end it is often very much appreciated by hostess and other guests alike. But that's part of another section of this book.

The point I want to make now is this: though some people have more stamina than others, no woman can look and feel her best and really be in top social form night after night if she's shortchanging herself on sleep. (The same is true of men, naturally.) I need the standard eight hours. You may need somewhat more or less. But whatever your sleep needs, it's important not to overlook them.

Smoking and Drinking and Why They're Bad for Your Looks

It used to be smart to smoke, but that was *ages* ago. Now it's much smarter not to.

As you know, smoking is just plain bad for you. It's been proven beyond a doubt that it makes you more vulnerable to a number of killer diseases. There is also the fact that the heavy smoker often has chronic bad breath—and that he or she is more and more looked upon as a kind of social nuisance, fouling the air in public places, and worst of all, at the dinner table. (Ever try to enjoy a meal in a restaurant with people at the next table blowing smoke your way?)

Smoking in the street is an ugly habit. More important, smoking seems to speed up the aging process of the skin. That's because it has a negative effect on the circulation, and good circulation is a must for good skin. Women who smoke seem to get more pronounced wrinkles, especially around the eyes (could it be from squinting through the nicotine haze?) and mouth. Smokers also wrinkle earlier in life.

It's interesting, I think, that some women who were only partially motivated to stop smoking when they were told it was bad for their health finally quit for good when they learned it's bad for their looks. Sometimes it seems the American Heart Association and the Cancer Society are approaching the problem all wrong. Maybe both organizations would have greater success with their antismoking campaigns if they placed heavier emphasis on the effects of smoking on physical appearance.

Heavy drinking, too, is bad for one's looks. Alcohol depletes the supply of moisture in the tissues. After a while, the woman who drinks even moderately—meaning two or three cocktails a day—may find her complexion getting progressively drier and duller-looking. Then, too, alcohol dilates the blood vessels. In time, some of the tiny vessels may burst. Apparently these tiny burst vessels are no threat to one's health, but the little red marks they leave are hardly attractive.

I don't smoke. I've never even tried it. The smell of other people's cigarettes was always enough to turn me off. As for drinking, I may have two or three glasses of white wine at dinner with friends—never more and never when I dine alone. I find the taste of what they call "hard liquor"—gin, vodka, whiskey, and so on—unpleasant, like the smell of smoke.

I'm not giving myself a pat on the back for being a nonsmoker and nondrinker. I'm certainly not depriving myself because of what smoking and drinking might do to my looks. It's just that neither habit appeals to me. In that way, I'm lucky. If they did appeal to me, I'd have problems. When I like something, I like it in a big way.

Earlier I mentioned my healthy habits. I love life. I want to feel good, I want to go on enjoying myself. So I try to take care of myself. I think that accounts for the fact that I can get by without a complicated, time-consuming beauty routine. It may also account for the look on people's faces when I tell them the ages of my children—twenty-seven, twenty-five, and twenty-two. That, and the fact that I don't fret about my appearance.

Upper and Downer People

There are beautiful women. There are attractive, interesting-looking women. And then there are women with sad, mad, sour, jealous written all over their faces.

Given the choice, we'd all prefer to be beautiful. Of course, that choice isn't open to any one of us. You're either born a Merle Oberon, a Babe Paley, or a Liz Taylor or you're not. But every woman can choose to be attractive, even if her features taken one by one are far from perfect.

To me, Gloria Guinness is the epitome of attractiveness and style. She's an up person, vibrant and alive. Her face positively radiates joie de vivre. Being with her, you can't help feeling good, more alive, yourself. In my opinion, Gloria's qualities are unique.

By contrast, there's a woman I know who, though physically attractive, is a complainer, a person consumed by jealousy. Her unhappiness and her pettiness are reflected in her face and she is not the beauty she could be. I run into her socially from time to time, but I'd just as soon not. She's a downer and it's easy to forget how beautiful she is.

Ugliness, I think, is a matter of choice. It usually has far less to do with the size and shape of the eyes, nose, and mouth than with the psychological state of being a downer.

Jealousy shows up on a face. Bitterness and resentment do too. I

In Acapulco with my friend Merle Oberon, one of the most beautiful women in the world . . . and also quite a bit more sensible about the sun than I am.

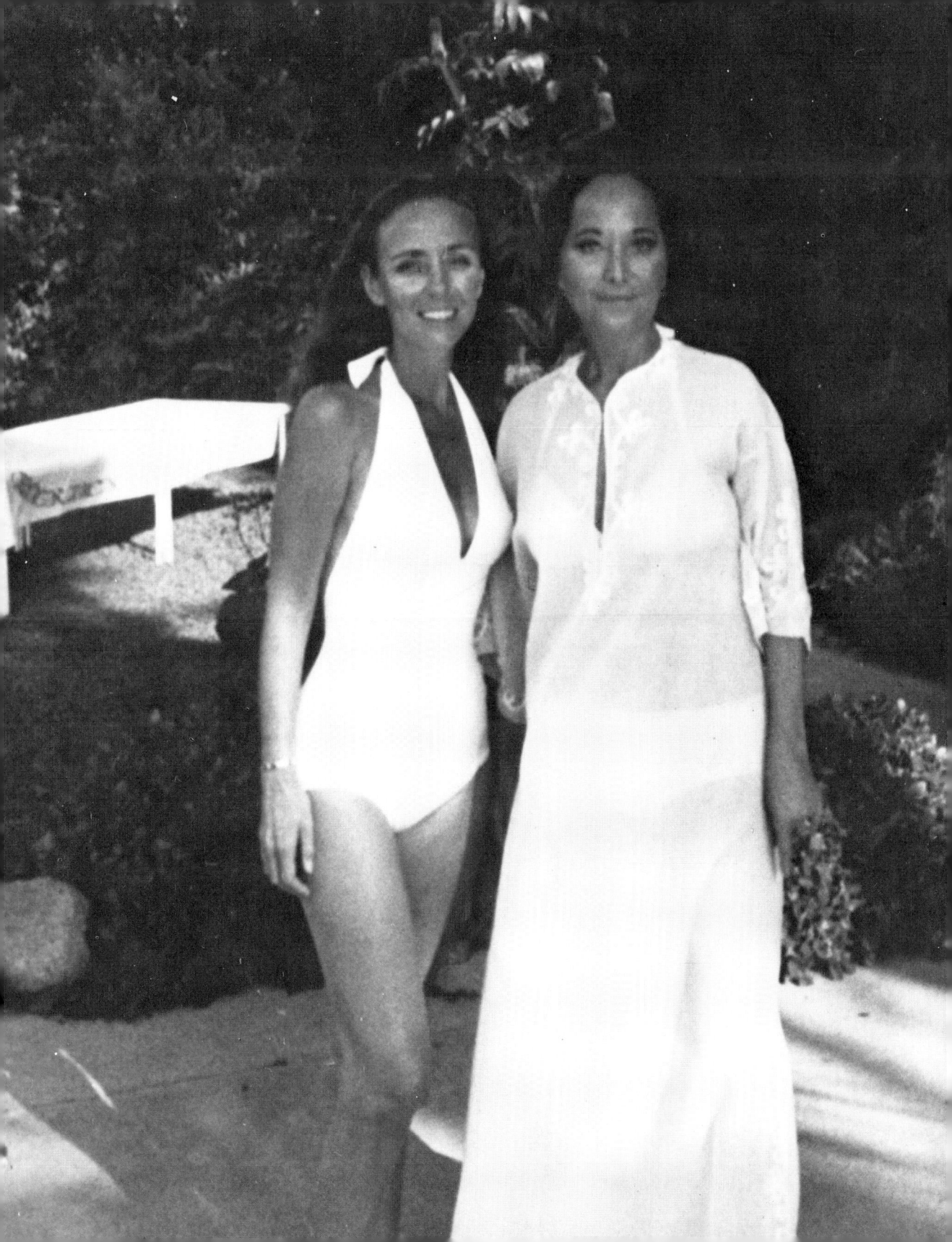

know women who are dreadfully unhappy with their husbands and always complaining about them. Yet they go on living with the men, using their husbands' money and prestige. That's fine, I guess. Or maybe they're masochistic and feel a need to put themselves and their husbands down. That's okay too, at least I'm not the one to criticize another person's feelings. Or maybe they think it's smart to advertise their unhappiness. What they don't seem to understand is that they're writing all that unhappiness into their faces. If they're really unhappy, and they really want the best for themselves, they could do themselves a favor and change the unhappy parts of their lives.

Boredom is another kind of unhappiness that shows up on a face. A woman whose days are empty and meaningless and who can't or won't find worthwhile creative outlets for her energies is rarely lovely to look at.

We're all entitled to our moods, of course. We can't help being sad or angry when things don't go the way we want them to. But there's no point in wallowing in misery or advertising it, especially to people who can't help us out anyway. I don't feel it's dishonest to grin and bear it, to put on a happy face. I've often found that someone else's response to my own attempts at cheerfulness helped pull me out of a blue mood.

I was talking on the phone the other day to Neil Walsh, the New York City commissioner of civic affairs and public events. He said, "Hello, Lyn, how are you?" I replied in an upbeat tone, "Why, fine, Neil. Great!" (The truth is, I'd just had a piece of bad news, but it didn't concern him and there was no reason to burden him with my problem. I'm glad I didn't.)

"You know," he said, "I must have made twenty phone calls today. And each time I said 'How are you?' I got nothing but moans and groans. I was beginning to feel grouchy myself, but I feel good now, talking to you."

And I felt better after talking to him.

What has all this to do with improving your looks? Only that being up is always attractive. Much, much more so than whining and complaining and being down. I really believe that one of the most important things any woman who wants to improve her looks can do is to cultivate an up frame of mind.

So much for generalities. It's time to be more specific.

Makeup: Finding What's Best for You

I'm going to assume that you wear makeup. Most American women do. Makeup is such a necessity to the women in this country that when money is tight, many would rather deprive themselves of food than go without lipstick. (It's true; I've seen the elaborate studies that prove it.)

I'm not sure what that says about our values, but there's no doubt that the right makeup, skillfully applied, can make any woman look more attractive.

It's interesting to me that though almost all of us wear makeup every day of our lives, many women are still mystified by it. It *can* be confusing. There are so many different kinds of products to choose from, in so many different formulations and colors, and there are new ones coming out each day. And then there's the fashion element. For a few years, eyes are in and lips are out. Then lips are in and eyes are out. Then it's the heavy, frankly made-up matte-finish look. Then the shiny, moist, natural look. And so on. You know it; there's a new one every season.

It becomes a lot less confusing when you stop thinking in terms of keeping up with fashion and achieving a series of different looks, and start concentrating on perfecting *a* look—the one that does the most for *you*.

Once you've found that best look, you can keep it for years, modifying it only somewhat with the seasons, the occasion, or when you discover a brand-new product that does wonders for you (though I must say I've worn the same basic makeup with only the slightest variations, summer and winter, day and night, since I was nineteen).

How do you find your best makeup look? That's another one of those questions that I can't answer specifically. What I can do is tell you how I arrived at mine and offer a few general guidelines that may *help* you find your own.

To begin with, I've always looked my best in the summer with a tan. I decided I wanted to keep that tawny sun-bronzed look all year round, even in the winter (*especially* in the winter) when my skin is much paler. I do it with makeup.

I tie my hair back, clean off my magnifying mirror, then go to work.

I start with a dark foundation, Revlon's Ultima II Creme Gel Sheer Coverage in Deep Copper Bronze. I squeeze a little into my right palm, take some on my fingertips, dot it on my cheeks, forehead, nose, and chin, and blend it in.

No, it doesn't match my skin tones. If I chose a makeup to match my skin, I'd end up looking pasty, and I don't want that.

Note: Trying to match your makeup to your skin tones is almost always a mistake. It may be *the* most common makeup mistake. Even women who want a pale, fragile look are better off with a foundation color that's a shade or two darker than their natural skin tones. Otherwise they run the risk of looking ashen or chalky.

But, you may be thinking to yourself, makeup that is so much darker than the natural skin tones *has* to look heavy and artificial. Not necessarily so. At least not with the kind of makeup I use. It's sheer, so sheer that my freckles show through. All it adds is color. There's none of the caked-on look you have to be careful of when you wear a heavier, more opaque makeup. (However, the woman who wants to hide minor skin imperfections wouldn't want to use such a transparent foundation; she probably should experiment with one that offers more coverage.)

Another reason why my makeup doesn't look artificial is that I apply it sparingly. I don't "paint walls" with it, as they say. And I'm careful to *blend it in.*

After the foundation, but before anything else, I lighten the area just under my eyes with something called Skin Paste by Janet Sartin. I use the "medium" shade. It comes in a little pot. I dot it on with a finger, starting at the inner corner of the eye and bringing it in a crescent to the other corner.

Next comes blusher. (If a dog is man's best friend, blusher is a woman's.) I use Revlon's Ultima II Blushing Creme in Deep Sienna. It's dark, almost brick color, and comes in a compact. It goes on with the fingers—one slash across the forehead, two on each cheek, going up toward the temples. Like the foundation, the blusher is blended in so that no one can tell where it begins or ends.

But don't think that's the end of it. Now I deepen my "tan" with Ultima II Ultra-Color Gelstick in Bronzelit Copper. It comes in a stick, like an oversized crayon. I stroke it across my forehead and on each cheek, then blend it in.

There's *more*. Over everything else goes Ultima II Sheer Radiance All-Over Face Color in Rich Bronze. It's a liquid flecked with gold. I dot it on my cheeks and forehead, then blend it in evenly. Completely transparent, all it adds is a nice golden sheen.

Now I'm ready to do my eyes. They're gray-green and I like to emphasize the green with a very pale green shadow. Ultima II Ultra-creme Eyeshadow in Silver Leaf, a light silvered green, is just right. I take some on my finger and—starting at the inner corner and going to the outer corner of each eye—apply it across the lid, close to the lashes. I bring a bit of color up to the tip of each eyebrow. Then I blend it in. Above the green, I add a stroke of Revlon's Natural Wonder Shiny Crayon Eye Shadow in Big Beige and *blend it* in.

Then eye liner. I use Ultima II Brush-on Cremeliner in Soft Black, which is better on me than a true black. It comes with a little brush. I wipe the excess off on a tissue first, then make a very fine line from the inner corner to the outer corner of each eye, as close to the lashes as possible. I don't finish up with an upward swoop as many women do. (I notice Diane von Furstenberg often draws an upward-pointing line and it looks just fine on her.)

Mascara is next. I use Revlon's Super-Rich Black Mascara. It goes on with a wand. I've found I can make my lashes look very full and long if I swoop it on the lashes of one eye a few times, then do the same with the other eye. Then a second coat for the first eye, which is almost dry by then, and a final second coat for the other eye.

The final step is lip gloss. The one I use is Lip Sartinizer by Janet Sartin. I apply it with my finger from a little pot. It's very shiny, but colorless.

Yes, I know, a fresh red mouth is the thing now (or is while I'm writing this). But I want my eyes to be the focal point of my face, and red lips would only tend to draw attention *away* from my eyes.

I'm sure you understand that I didn't give this blow-by-blow description of my makeup so that you could run out and buy all the products I use and apply them exactly as I do. I wanted to get the idea across that you can do a lot with makeup—more perhaps than you ever thought you could. I didn't just stumble onto the idea of wearing a foundation, two kinds of blusher, a transparent golden sheen, etc. Nobody told me to use these products or how to apply them. Not at all. I knew the look I wanted to achieve and I kept on experimenting until I got it. You can do the same.

It's important to add that I don't look any more "made-up" than women who use only one or two things on their faces—I may even look less made-up because I'm so careful to blend everything in. The final effect is less makeup, more slightly sunburned glow.

Some people don't believe I wear anything but eye makeup. Even people I know quite well come up to me and comment on my fabulous winter "tan." When I tell them no, I haven't been to Palm Beach and I don't sit under a sunlamp, they look skeptical. Usually I don't argue. People believe what they want to believe. But once when I wanted to prove my point to a woman I know, I wiped a tissue across my face. She gasped—literally—when she saw all the brick-colored makeup on the tissue.

A Few Basic Makeup Dos and Don'ts

Always start with a clean face. You've probably found out that makeup can't do all the nice things it could if it's applied over old makeup and grime.

I clean my face by scrubbing it with soap lathered into a washcloth, a practice many beauty experts say is too harsh for a woman's skin. All I can say is it's not too harsh for *my* skin or I'd have noticed it by now since I've *always* washed my face that way. Soap and gentle friction from the washcloth do an excellent job of removing grime, oil, and old makeup, along with the topmost layer of dead skin cells that can make a complexion look dull and lifeless.

My complexion, don't forget, is oily. It can take rougher treatment than skin that is dry or sensitive.

Soap and washcloth cleaning may not be the best choice for you if your skin is normal or dry. In that case, it might be better to use a mild soap and lather it on with your hands. Or, if your skin is dry, try a "washable" cleansing lotion. These lotions are thin, creamy-white emulsions that are less drying than soap but are easily rinsed off with water, so there's no greasy residue. (Many of these products have the words "milk" or "milky cleanser" in their names.) A washable lotion is often a good choice even for *very* dry skin—better than cleansing creams which, despite their names, don't do a very good job of removing makeup and grime.

Use a foundation shade that is darker than your natural skin tone. I can't emphasize this too much. I know women who've tried to match their skin tones with every conceivable *kind* of makeup and been dissatisfied. A simple switch to darker makeup worked wonders.

Don't hesitate to experiment with—and wear—a variety of different products all at once. But apply them all sparingly. Don't "paint walls." Within a matter of hours, gobs of heavy makeup start to look cakey and cracked. Smile lines and any little wrinkles you have around the eyes or on your forehead will be emphasized.

In general, try to use the sheerest makeup possible. If your skin is good, try one of the transparent foundations. If it's not so good, you'll probably want to go on to something heavier. But keep in mind that although makeup can even out slight discolorations and camouflage little imperfections, it won't hide pimples or wrinkles. If it's applied too heavily, it may even call attention to them.

Be careful to blend in foundation and blusher very thoroughly so that there are no harsh lines of demarcation. Bring foundation down to just slightly under the jaw, then blend. There's no need to wear makeup on your neck. It will only rub off on your collar.

Play with color all you like, but remember that certain very vivid hues around the eyes—bright pink, yellow, purple, and green, for example—which might look well under some lighting conditions may be harsh and garish under others. Be careful with them.

Unless you're very young, a sharp, heavy black line around the eye is cheap-looking. It also tends to make the lid look heavy and the eye itself smaller rather than larger.

False eyelashes, too, tend to look cheap unless they're trimmed to a reasonable length and thickness. They also must be perfectly applied. (I've never liked the look of false eyelashes so I've never even tried to wear them. I'd rather thicken and lengthen my lashes with mascara.)

Read the cosmetic ads in the magazines to find out about new products and take a good look at the models in *Vogue* and *Bazaar* to see what they're wearing on their faces. But remember that the models in the advertisements and on the editorial pages are made up for photography, not real life. What looks great in a photograph may look positively bizarre strolling down Main Street at high noon.

On bad days when you have a cold or weren't able to get enough sleep the night before, reach for the eyedrops. Lately I've been using a product called Clear Eyes, made by Abbott Laboratories. A drop or two in each eye seems to take away the red, tired look. You may also want to give yourself an extra helping of color—more blusher, in other words. It may not work for you, but it always makes me look and feel better. At least give it a try.

And now let's talk about hair.

Your Hair and How to Find the Best Way to Wear It

As you know, I'm convinced that each woman has a best look. That goes for the clothes she wears, as well as her makeup—and of course, her hair. Some women have a repertoire of different looks, but there's always *one* best look. Finding that one best look and then polishing it—that's what establishing a unique physical style is all about.

Long hair is definitely my best look. I've had short hair once in my life, but I'm convinced that long hair is more flattering for *me*. It's become an integral part of my personal style, and I'll wear my hair long until my mirror—not my hairdresser, not my friends, not the man in my life—but my *mirror* tells me it's time for a change. I don't care if it looks the same day after day and year after year. If I *like* the way it looks—day after day and year after year—isn't that the important thing?

Strange, though, the way some people try to prod others into changing. "But, Lyn, don't you know curls are in?" say some of my well-meaning friends. Or, "But, Lyn, everyone is wearing short hair now." I'm not sure what motivates these comments. I certainly don't need to be told who's wearing what. But I do appreciate their concern. What they don't seem to understand is that they don't have to live with my hair; *I* do.

I mean that part about "living with my hair" quite literally. Long hair not only looks best on me, it's easiest for me to live with. You see, my feeling is that no matter how sensational a certain hairstyle might look, it would be all wrong for me if I had to spend great amounts of time and energy keeping it up.

As it is, my hair requires only a shampoo and blow-dry once a week in the winter—more often in the summer. For this I go to Marc Sinclaire at Elizabeth Arden. He's a wonderfully talented man who works quickly and knows just how to handle my hair. I find it's much easier and more convenient to have him do it than to do it myself.

However, I can always take care of my own hair if need be. I never go to a hairdresser when I'm out of town, except when I'm in Paris. (Then I go to Alexandre.) Instead, I wash my hair in the bathtub with Johnson & Johnson No More Tears baby shampoo. It's mild and doesn't dry my hair. I like it so much that I always make sure that Marc has a bottle of No More Tears on hand at the salon.

Aside from lots of brushing, and having it trimmed once a year or so, that's about all the special care my hair ever gets. (Oh, yes. Once I had a rather interesting treatment to get rid of split ends. It was done in a salon and involved quickly singeing the end of each hair with a match. The smell was awful, like burnt chicken feathers. And

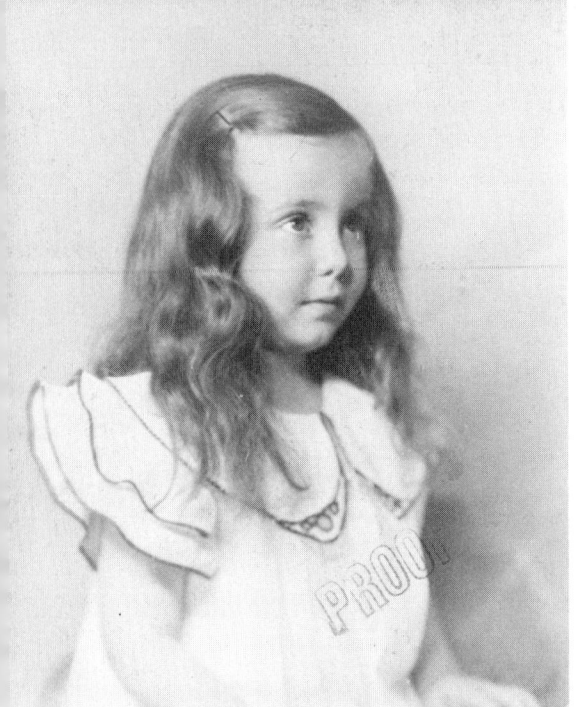

Long hair was always my best look... at four (PHOTO: L. DEE);

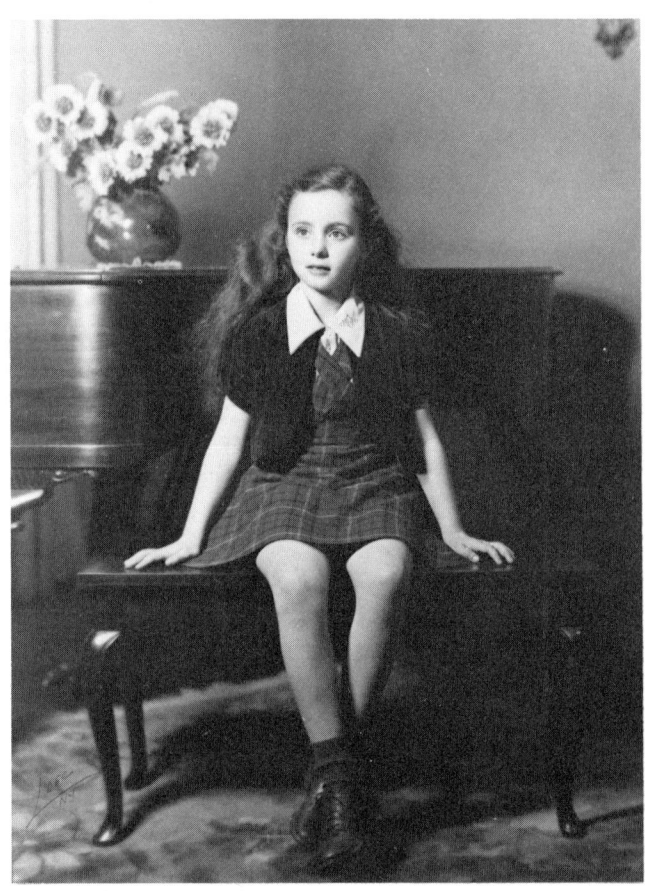

...at nine (I never did learn to play the piano) (PHOTO: L. DEE);

...and today. (PHOTO: WWD)

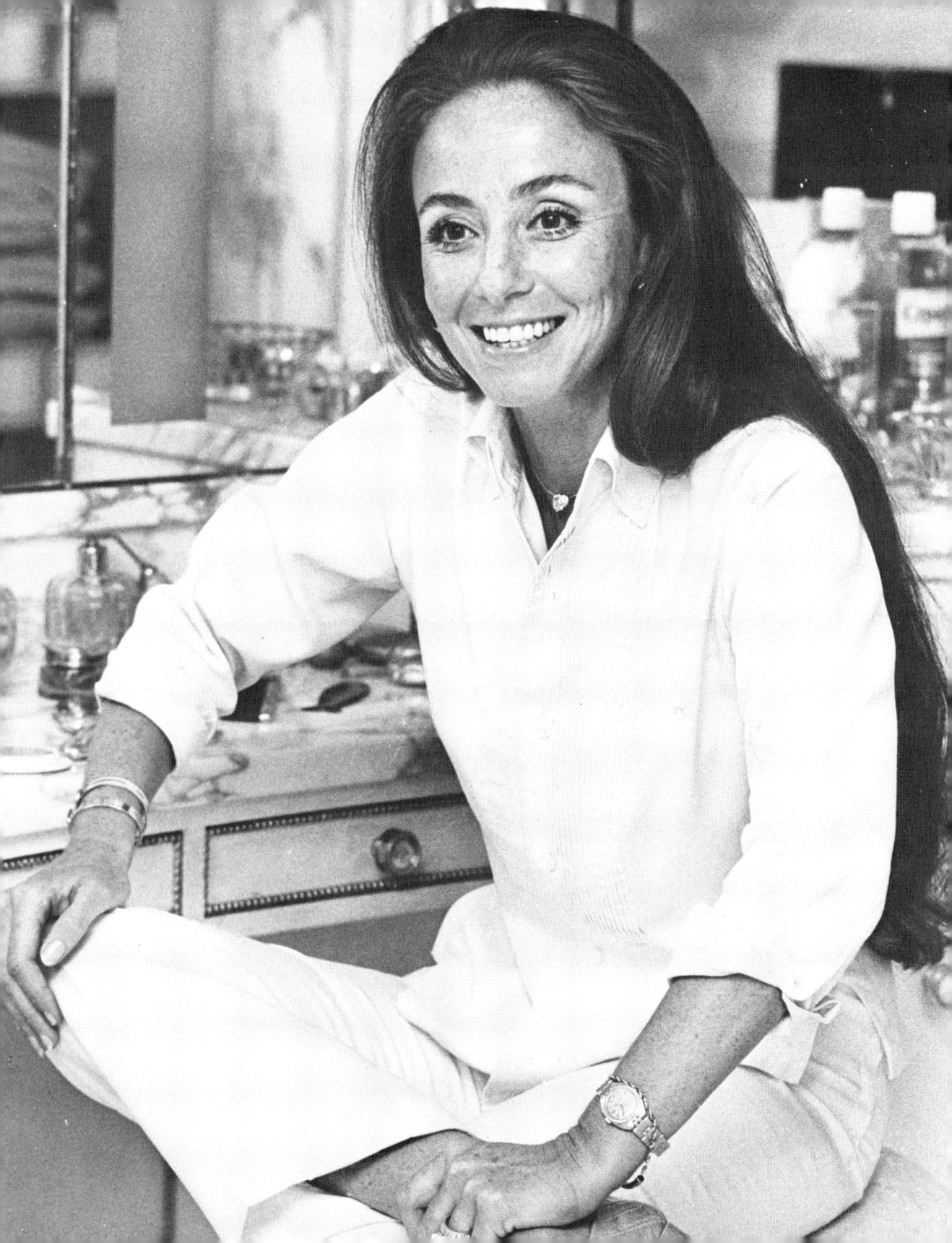

I didn't think the results were worth the time and money. So it's a process I don't recommend. Trimming off the ends in the conventional way, with scissors, seems like a much better solution to the split ends problem.)

I know I'm lucky to have good hair. It's thick and strong now that I've stopped pulling it back with a rubber band. (Rubber bands were breaking my hair; now I use a ponytail holder, or fasten it with a single giant hairpin.) But long hair isn't for everyone. The last thing in the world I want to encourage you to do is to try and solve your hair problems by wearing your hair, and treating it, as I do mine. My hairstyle and the way I care for my hair simply may not work for you. (Remember, you have to live with your hair, not I.)

I do have a few suggestions that might help you in finding, and maintaining, your own best hair look.

First, work with what you have. I think this is the most important tip of all. It applies across the board to almost every aspect of beauty, but especially to hair.

Unless you're willing to spend an awful lot of time and energy fussing with your hair, you're better off with a hairstyle suited to your particular kind of hair rather than trying to suit your hair to a particular style.

For example, if your hair is naturally straight and smooth, you (and/or your hairdresser) will have to work hard at achieving and maintaining a very curly look. You *could* have a perm, but a permanent tends to dry the hair, and then, unless you keep on reperming, there's that bothersome growing-out stage. Or, you could set it on rollers yourself, or have it set, every day or every other day. But that can be terribly time-consuming and most of us have better things to do.

If your hair is wavy, curly, or frizzy and you want a smoother look, you can always have it straightened. But again, the chemical process can be hard on your hair, the results are only temporary and never quite identical to the real thing—naturally silky, straight hair.

It makes much better sense to accept your hair as it is. To work with it, instead of against it. To make your hair—whether it's straight, wavy, curly, or a marvelous halo of frizz—a kind of trademark, the starting point of your own personal style.

As for color, again, stay pretty close to what you were born with. You already have a personal "color scheme." Nature gave it to you and nature makes very few mistakes. Eyes, skin tones, hair, and yes, even eyebrows, are just naturally harmonious. To change one element usually throws the others off key. And to get everything back into harmony again may mean making a host of other changes.

For example, the born brunette who bleaches her hair a light blonde usually has to have her eyebrows lightened too if she wants a natural look. She may also need to modify her skin tones with heavy makeup, since the dark olive skin that often goes along with being a born brunette clashes with blonde hair.

The natural blonde who dyes her hair dark brown may need to make those same changes in reverse in order to make her new brunette look convincing. And the woman who goes from blonde or brunette to red hair, or from red hair to blonde or brunette, has to make other kinds of changes.

It can get to be rather complicated. Worse, the real natural you gets lost beneath all those changes.

I've always suspected that one of the main reasons women make drastic changes in the color of their hair is because they want to look more like someone they admire.

A few years ago the question was "Do blondes have more fun?" Women went Brigitte-Bardot-blonde to find out. Audrey Hepburn was a big thing too. Now it's the Farrah Fawcett-Majors blonde and the Ali McGraw brunette. We all need heroes or heroines: people to look up to because of their courage and strength of character, their ingenuity and warmth. Emulating the good qualities of others helps us become better people ourselves. But trying to model yourself physically on another human being doesn't work. At best, you can turn yourself into a reasonably good facsimile. But why be a facsimile when you can be an original *you*?

Making a *slight* change in the color of your hair is something else again. When you add a few subtle streaks or highlights of gold or chestnut or copper, or tone your hair a shade or two darker for added drama, you're not altering your whole physical identity. You're not throwing your natural color scheme off balance. You're enhancing the best of what you already have.

How to Choose a Hairstyle

Now, what about the actual hairstyle itself? How do you decide which of the hundreds of different ways you could wear your hair is the best one for you? Obviously, you can't try and live with them all. Some of the following considerations may help you narrow the field down to three or four possible choices.

1. *How big are you?* How big is your body? Your head? Your face? You may be surprised that these particular questions come first. Perhaps you never thought of your size in connection with choosing a hairstyle. But the relationship is important.

Let me explain. Hair shouldn't just sit there on the top of your head looking decorative. It's part of your total look and it either works or it doesn't work with the rest of you. In general, the bigger your body, head, and face, the more hair you need for balance. The big woman with a very tiny, short hairstyle risks looking like a pinhead—even if that very same hairstyle "flatters" her face. And skinning all the hair back from the face doesn't make a big face look smaller, doesn't make large features appear to be more delicate. It only throws large face and features into greater relief.

Small people, on the other hand, tend to look top-heavy when their hair is piled high or worn massed around their faces, while very small features tend to get lost when a lot of hair is worn teased and close to the face.

2. *How do you live?* The Olympic swimmer definitely needs a wash-and-wear hairstyle. Most of the rest of us don't. Still, factors such as where you live, your activities, and the general pace of your life are important considerations when choosing a hairstyle.

If you live where it's quite warm all year round, you'll naturally be uncomfortable unless you wear your hair either very short, or long enough so that you can hike it up and off your neck into a ponytail or braid. If your life is filled with parties and formal dinners and balls, a breezy, casual style won't be right for you unless you or your hairdresser can easily convert it to a more sophisticated, dressed-up look. If you're on a tight budget, any gimmicky, tricky cut is to be avoided, since you'll need to keep going back to the salon every month or six weeks to keep it shaped up properly.

3. *What about age?* My feeling is that too many women give too much consideration to their age when choosing a hairstyle. I've heard women in their forties and even in their thirties say they'd love to wear a particular style, but they feel they're "too old" for it.

That's nonsense! There are women in their seventies who look marvelous in a close-cropped head-hugging "little boy" hairstyle, and others who look absolutely smashing in a smooth, turned-under style well past shoulder-length. (I've also seen the way some women suddenly aged considerably when they switched to a hairstyle that they—or their hairdressers—deemed more "appropriate" to their years.)

A hairstyle might be wrong for you for any number of reasons, but age probably isn't one of them. Like wearing lace-up granny shoes, one of the surest ways to *add* years to your looks is to settle on a hairstyle because you feel it's appropriate to your age.

4. *Consider the classics.* Contrived, tricky haircuts will come and go, but a few styles—simple, elegant, easy to wear—will be with us always. They are:

*Long hair of any type or texture, pulled back, and folded or gathered into a chignon or twist.

*Longish straight hair, worn silky smooth "Alice in Wonderland" or "Cleopatra" style, with or without bangs. (With the ends turned under, this style becomes a pageboy.)

*Frizzy, curly, or wavy hair cut in all-over layers, worn either very short, like a little helmet, or longer and fuller—depending on which is more flattering.

These are the classics—never dated, always appropriate, always "right." When you're choosing a hairstyle, it may help to start out by thinking in terms of one of them.

How to Care for Your Hair

Good hair care is such a common-sensical matter that I'm always amazed that so many beauty books devote so many pages to the obvious.

BRUSHING: Hair should be brushed frequently with a good natural-bristle hairbrush. (Nylon bristles are sharp and squared off at the ends and can damage the hair.) Brushing removes loose dirt and dandruff. It also stimulates the oil glands. Therefore, hair that tends to be oily will look and feel oilier still if it's brushed *too* often and *too* vigorously. (That doesn't mean you shouldn't brush at all if your hair is oily; only that you should brush less than the old standard hundred strokes a day. Instead, brush just enough to "freshen" your hair. Then stop.)

Here's a good tip: if your hair is very long, brush it in sections. First, brush all over from the scalp to about six inches from the scalp. Then, with one hand grasping a section of hair firmly at the six-inch "line," brush from there to the ends. (Continue in sections until all your hair has had a good going-over with the brush.) Brushing with one hand while "anchoring" your hair with the other reduces the pull on the roots. As a result, fewer individual hairs are yanked out and there's less breakage.

Short hair or long, the final step in brushing is to bend down, flipping your hair forward, and brush hair up from the nape of the neck.

NOTE: Hair is weakest when it's wet, so never brush right after shampooing. Comb it out *gently* instead.

COMBING: Choose a hard rubber comb, one with widely spaced teeth. Never pull or yank through tangles; that kind of rough treatment breaks the hair. Instead, you can unsnarl stubborn knots by first moistening your comb with a dab of cream rinse, then unsnarling the tangle—gently—starting from the ends of the hair and working up toward the scalp.

SHAMPOOING: It stands to reason that oily hair will need more frequent shampooing than dry hair, and that either kind will need to be washed more often in warm weather or when participation in active sports causes your scalp to perspire freely. As for what kind of shampoo to use, the gentler the better. (That's why I prefer baby shampoo for myself.) Experiment until you find a product that you like. Many brand-name shampoos come in several formulations—one for oily hair, one for dry or damaged hair, one for color-treated hair, etc. Start out with the one best suited to your particular hair type. But don't forget, everyone's hair is different and it could be that a shampoo for dry or damaged hair (usually the gentlest in any manufacturer's line) works best for you, even though your hair might best be described as "normal."

CREAM RINSES AND CONDITIONERS: I don't use them. They tend to make my hair softer and "limper" than I like. However, if your hair is very dry and unmanageable, or baby-fine and without body, some kind of shampoo follow-up is probably a good idea. The shelves of any reasonably well-stocked pharmacy or department store are bursting with after-shampoo products labeled for every conceivable type of hair and hair problem. Once again, experiment until you find one that gives you good results.

HAIR DRYERS: The blow dryer is a marvelous invention. If you don't own one, get one. In the summer when I play tennis, I use a blow dryer constantly. Just in case one breaks down, I have two.

If you're not sure how to use the contraption even after reading the manufacturer's instruction booklet, ask your hairdresser for a few pointers. (Incidentally, if my hairdresser couldn't or wouldn't explain at least some of the tricks of the trade, I'd find a new one!)

One thing to keep in mind about the blow dryer. It can dry and ultimately damage your hair if you use it too often at very high heat. Though it may take slightly longer, using the blow dryer (or any dryer) on the "warm" setting is much kinder to your hair.

HAIR SPRAY: This is another product I hardly ever use, mainly because of the way I wear my hair; it's *supposed* to move. However, if the success of your hairstyle depends on its holding a certain line, then hair spray can be a big help. Use the kind with the gentlest "hold" and spray it on lightly.

How to Choose a Good Hairdresser

Some of the top hairdressers are a little bit like fashion designers. They have good years when, because they've created a new look or because they've been taken up by the editors of a magazine or a group of trend-setting women (or because they've written a best-selling book), they achieve "superstar" status. Then, they fade into (relative) obscurity—often to be rediscovered and back in the limelight again a few years later.

I don't mean to knock any particular hairdresser. It probably isn't possible for anyone to become a superstar without demonstrating real talent. But I don't think it follows that just because hairdresser X is hot at the moment, he is therefore the hairdresser for you. In fact, I can think of at least one good reason why he may be the worst possible choice.

Suppose hairdresser X suggests short, curly hair? Obviously, there's no problem if that's what you yourself had in mind. But what if you wanted something different? It takes a fairly strong personality not to be intimidated (perhaps "persuaded" is a better word) by a superstar. It's easy to feel he *must* have an insight into what's best for you simply because he *is* a superstar. I think you have to resist this feeling, and if you're uncomfortable about what he suggests, you have to speak up. Otherwise, you may find yourself an hour and a half later with a hairstyle you'll be hating for months afterward.

Or, perhaps superstar hairdresser X made his reputation with a certain "trademark" haircut. Again, there's no problem if you truly want to wear his trademark. But if you don't, you may be better off going to someone else. I've heard of instances where a hairdresser just wasn't interested in doing hair any way but *his* way.

Of course, all superstars aren't so temperamental. Many of them, probably even most, are exceptionally talented people whose primary concern is that their clients leave the salon looking and feeling marvelous. Superstar or not, that should be the goal of every good hairdresser.

How do you find and work with a good hairdresser?

1. Obviously, one way to locate a good hairdresser is to ask around among your friends and acquaintances—especially the ones with great-looking hair. You might even ask for a recommendation from a woman you've just met at a party, perhaps, or a dinner. (Let her know how much you like her hair; she'll probably be delighted to tell you who her hairdresser is. If she'd rather not tell you or if she just shrugs and says, "Oh, no one special," don't press her further. Some women are very possessive of their hairdressers and are extremely reluctant to give out this kind of information.)

2. If no one you know has a good hairdresser (or if no one is willing to talk), keep an eye on *Vogue, Bazaar,* and *Town & Country.* These magazines all occasionally mention hairdressers in various areas across the country who do excellent work.

3. If you're getting nowhere with the first two suggestions, and you want a hairdresser *now,* phone the store with the best fashion reputation in town. Ask for an appointment with the person who does the best _____ (fill in the blank for whatever you want to have done —cutting, coloring, etc.). Now suppose you've located a hairdresser and made an appointment. When you arrive, tell him how you feel about your hair as it is, what you like about it and what you don't. Then listen to his suggestions. Have him shape and style your hair, but don't make any drastic changes just yet. Assuming you're happy with his work, this may be the beginning of a beautiful, long-lasting relationship. But only if: (a) He gently suggests rather than forcefully tries to persuade you to make changes you're hesitant about. Let him tell you what he wants to do and why, but if his suggestions sound like orders, you may be better off with someone else. (b) He tells you —or shows you—how to take care of your own hair. He gives you

pointers on how to use the blow dryer, how to set your hair, how to back-comb it for more fullness. (Marc Sinclaire, my hairdresser, is a great teacher. Among other things, he taught me to make a chignon. My hair is so long, my arms are falling off when I try to do it myself. But now I can do a fairly good job if I have to.)

If your hairdresser doesn't volunteer this kind of information, for heaven's sake *ask* him. I'd think twice about continuing with someone who seemed too busy or too bored to share some of his professional expertise.

It also helps if your hairdresser is the kind who, no matter how many other clients he has, focuses exclusively on you when you're with him. That means he doesn't run off for coffee or to chat with another hairdresser or client during *your* time. (Emergencies arise, of course, and you should try to be understanding when they do.)

Finally, and this may not seem as important to you as it is to me, I'd be wary of the hairdresser who is a busybody. I have friends whose hairdressers have passed along to them the most outrageous information about other clients. Well, there's every reason to believe that the hairdresser who gossips about others to you won't hesitate to gossip about you to others. Be guided accordingly. (In defense of the hairdresser, I have to add that many women use the man who does their hair as father-confessor or shrink. Hairdressers are only human. When handed a big, juicy piece of gossip, most of them want to share it. One woman I know uses her hairdresser as a messenger, giving him such assignments as finding out why another client has been cool to her. Hairdressers are people with work to do. If they're going to do it well, they shouldn't have to be bothered with such things.)

A Few Words about Teeth

Teeth, I think, are greatly underrated in the beauty department. The same grown-up women who spend fortunes on their children's teeth often forget that their own teeth, too, need looking after. Many of the

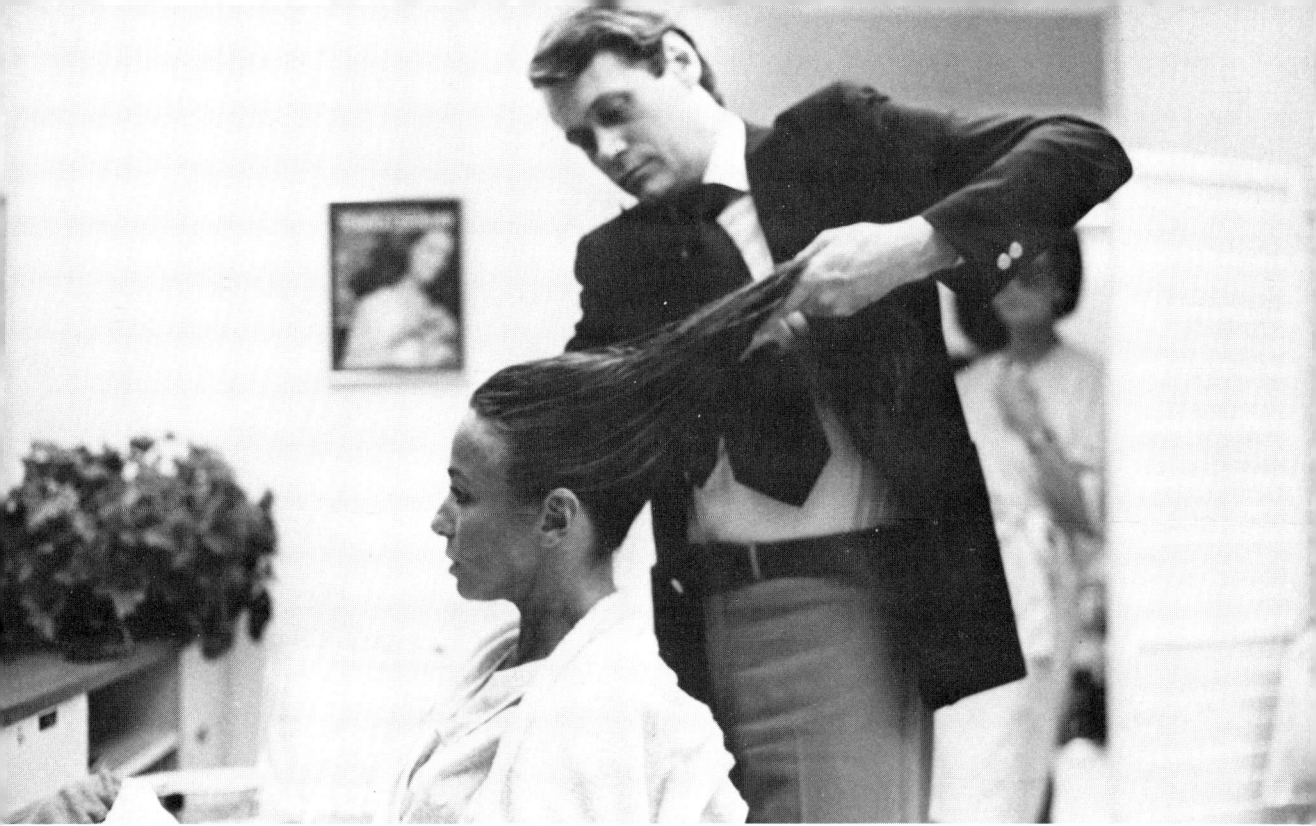

Marc Sinclaire of Elizabeth Arden combing my wet hair before blow-drying it. (PHOTO: JEFFREY SHERESKY)

same women who pay very careful attention to all other aspects of their appearance—who are meticulous about their hair, go on a diet at the first sign of overweight, exercise faithfully, and learn to apply makeup with the deft touch of a professional—overlook their teeth completely. When they open their mouths, it's a shock. (Except that people with bad teeth usually know it and don't open their mouths if they can help it.)

I know, going to the dentist is not one of life's most pleasant experiences. Even if your dentist is painless and a wonderful old friend, as is mine, Dr. Maurice Saklad, clinical professor at New York University, it's hardly a fun way to spend an afternoon. Pleasant or not, if you really want to make the most of your looks, you must take care of your teeth.

Modern dentistry being what it is, there's no reason why anyone needs to walk around with an unsightly mouthful of teeth. Very crooked teeth can be straightened—and should be—no matter what

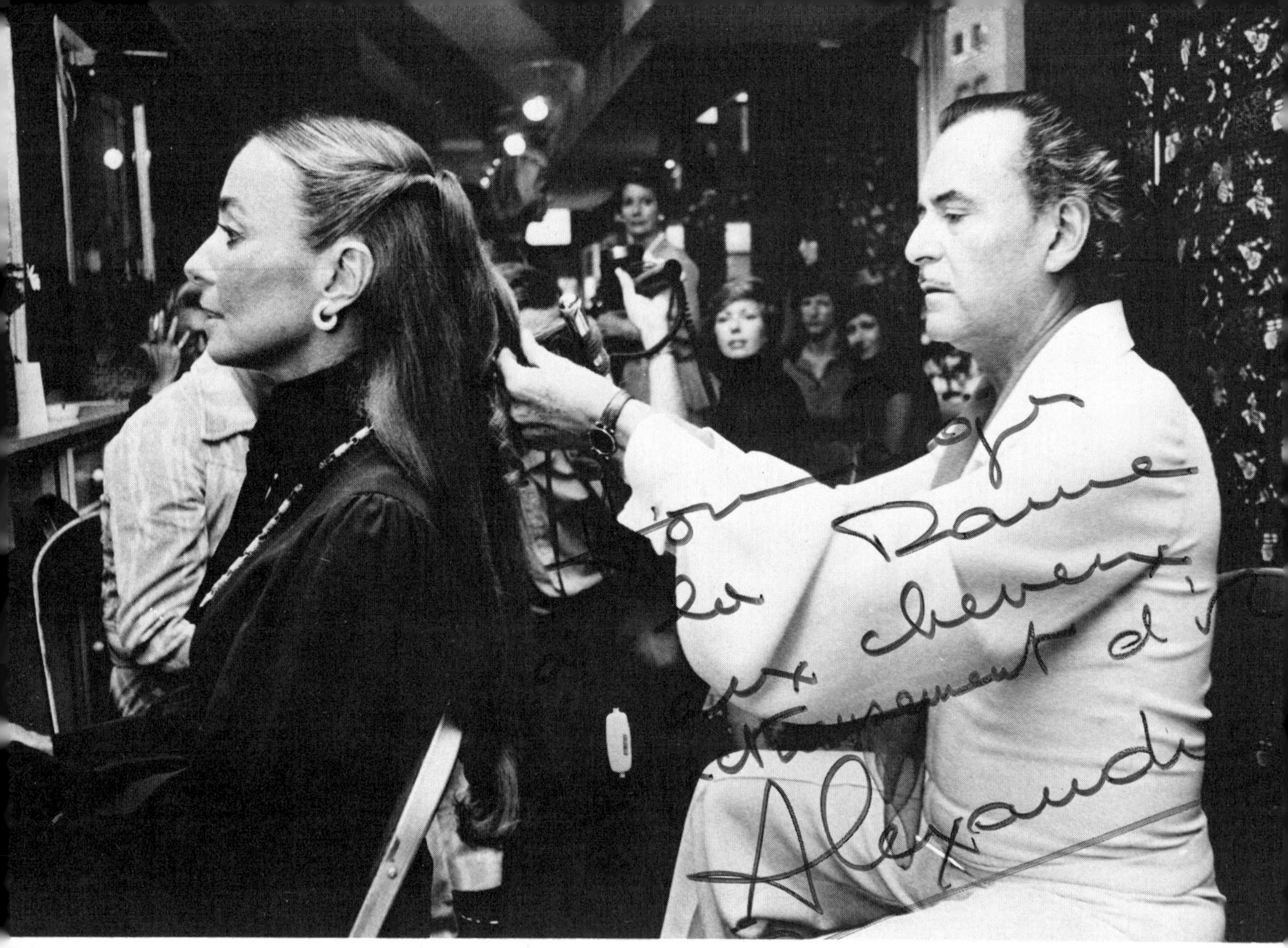

In Paris, Alexandre does my hair. He inscribed this 1975 photograph *Homage à la Dame aux cheveux d'or*. ("Praise to the woman with the golden hair.")

One of the working sketches for which he's so well known.

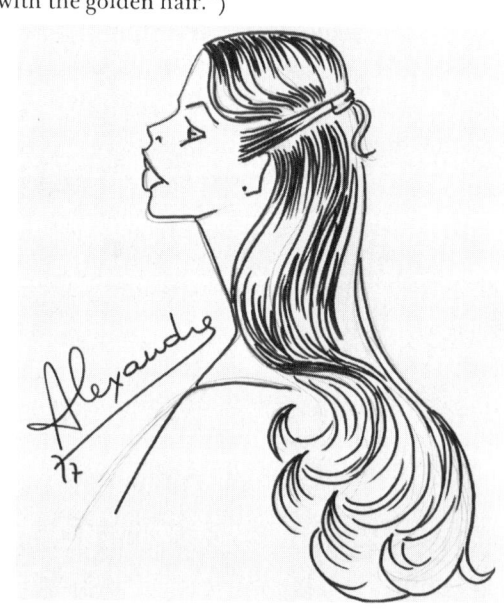

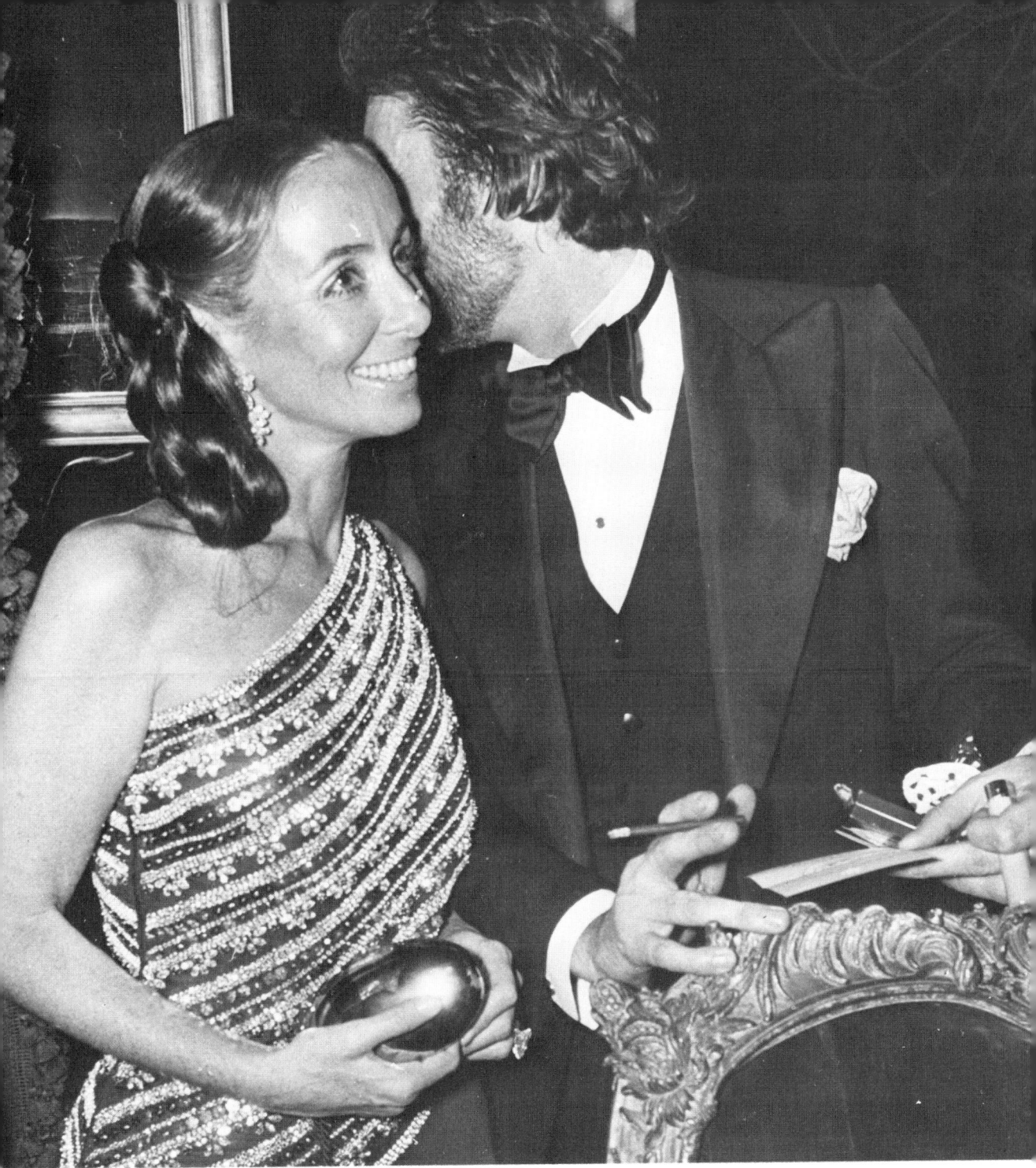

For a party in Paris given by Baron Alexis de Rede, Alexandre braided my hair to one side, to balance the one-shoulder Galanos dress. The man telling me the big secret is André Oliver, whose new menswear boutique on East Fifty-seventh Street is a smashing success. (PHOTO: REGINALD GRAY/WWD)

your age. Decayed teeth can be repaired. And if all else fails, you can always have your teeth capped.

As for the cost, yes, getting your mouth into good shape may be an expensive undertaking. But no more expensive, in many cases, than two weeks in the West Indies. Or a fox jacket. If I had to choose, I'd opt for a good-looking mouth any day. Having a healthy mouth isn't only for good looks—it insures the health of the rest of your body, too.

Fragrance: How to Choose It and Wear It

I love perfume. I always have. My favorite fragrance is Bal à Versailles and I wear it all the time. Though I don't put those special little pads soaked with fragrance on my light bulbs as Françoise de la Renta does (a wonderful idea—maybe I *should* start doing it), my apartment does tend to have a rather distinct air of Bal à Versailles about it—mainly because *I'm* there, and I wear a lot of it. My children tell me they always know if I've recently entered or left the house because a trace of my fragrance lingers on in the elevator.

I like that. I like the idea that a particular fragrance reminds people of me. Even cabdrivers remember me by my fragrance. (It's true. Once I got into a cab, the driver inhaled deeply, then turned around and said, "I remember you, the lady with the perfume." Another cabdriver said he wanted to drive me around for nothing, he liked my fragrance so much.) That's why I don't change my perfume. I wear it night and day, summer and winter. Perfume, to me, is much more than something to make me smell good. It's become another aspect—and a very important one—of my personal style.

It seems to me that any woman who wants to cultivate a style of her own should give some thought to selecting a fragrance. When she finds one that she loves, she should wear it. Not just on special evenings, not just in the company of certain people, but always, everywhere. Then it becomes as much her as the way she walks, talks, and signs her name.

Which of the hundreds of different fragrances on the market will become your signature perfume? Like so many other things that fall into the realm of personal style, you can't leave the choice to someone else. *You* have to live with your selection, so you have to love it. You probably already have two or three favorites, but if none of them seems quite right, then go out and do a little experimenting at the perfume counters of the largest, best-stocked department store in your area. There you will find sample bottles of fragrance for you to test.

Don't be shy or stingy about it. Spray generously. Wait a while—say five minutes or so—to give the alcohol a chance to evaporate. What's left is the perfume essence itself, which by now has reacted with your own particular skin chemistry.

Now breathe in the scent. Is it heavy or light, warm or cool, sparkling or soft, flowery, lemony, musky? Is it spicy, with a suggestion of cinnamon, clove, or ginger? Does it smell like a forest after a spring rain? Does it remind you of grandma's sachet? A cedar chest? A sandalwood box, or what?

Since most people are not professional "noses" (that's what they call the men and women who earn their livings creating and testing new perfumes) and can't file away a particular scent in their minds and recall it at will, it might help to jot down in a little notebook the name and your immediate impressions of each fragrance you test. You might even rate it in terms of how much you like it. Five stars for something you adore, a minus star for a fragrance that turns you off.

It's not a good idea to try to test more than two fragrances at a time. The untrained nose is easily confused. And anyway, you only have two arms to test with. Unless you wash away every last trace of a previously tested fragrance, you won't get an accurate reading of the next one you spray on.

If you're lucky, you'll fall in love with one of the first three or four fragrances you test. But don't count on it. It may take a while before you find one you like well enough to make it your signature. In any event, keep some of the following considerations in mind when you make a final decision.

1. Your signature fragrance should be versatile enough for day and night, summer and winter. Think twice about choosing an intense musky or *cloyingly* sweet floral scent. Either could be too heavy and "overpowering" to wear in warm weather.

2. Fragrance is not to be hoarded. If it's going to be worn and appreciated at all, it should be used *liberally*. (I'll explain how and why later.) Obviously then, your signature perfume should be affordable. If it turns out that the fragrance of your preference is in the $115-an-ounce range, and you can't spend that much on perfume, ask the salesperson to suggest something similar but less costly. (Some of the more expensive French perfumes have been "copied" by American manufacturers. The copies are not identical, of course, but they often capture the essential "spirit" of the originals.) Or you could use a cologne version of the perfume.

At the same time, I want to warn you away from very cheap perfume, which tends to smell . . . well . . . *cheap.*

3. Think twice about choosing a fragrance because you love it on one of your friends. It won't smell the same on you. Denise Hale always wears Jungle Gardenia by Tuvache and I adore it on her. No matter where I am, if she's anywhere nearby, I know it because of her fragrance. It doesn't smell the same on anyone else. It certainly doesn't smell the same on me. Years ago, inspired by her, I ran out to Saks for some Jungle Gardenia. The first time I wore it at home, the children, who were little then, told me it smelled like "all the monkeys had come out of the trees." I still don't know what they meant, but it wasn't good.

Which brings us to the best test of all. If you like a fragrance, and if you get compliments when you wear it, it's the right fragrance for you.

As for wearing perfume, I'm always amused when I see women

dabbing it on daintily from the bottle, putting a dot of it behind each ear, another dot at the crook of each elbow, and a final dot on each wrist. I know why they do it that way. All the magazines and beauty books point out that wrists, elbows, and behind the ears are "pulse points." They say that fragrance when applied to the pulse points is somehow warmed and intensified.

It's true. However, you don't get much mileage out of such a small amount of perfume dabbed on with a finger. After an hour or so, no one knows it's there. It's wasted.

It's much better to get an atomizer and spray it on all over—your neck, your chest and stomach, your shoulders, arms, and legs too. Do this just after your shower or bath but before getting into your clothes. And don't be afraid that the fragrance will be too strong. It won't be. It *will* last from morning to night, or bath time, and you'll be enveloped in a delicious, subtle aura of scent. People will know you're there.

A few more words about fragrance. From time to time I've mentioned that I prefer a certain bath or hair product because it's unscented, or only very delicately scented. There's a good reason for this. Heavily scented products often "clash" with a perfume. And what's the point of carefully choosing and wearing a signature scent if it's going to get mixed up with (and maybe even lost under) a host of other scents?

I also want to smell the same all over. Some shampoos, for example, have a lovely, appealing scent, but I don't want my hair to smell one way and the rest of me another. It's the same with body lotions, creams, and talcs.

If you're going to spend good money on perfume, it makes sense to underplay fragrance in the other products you use.

Finally, some women shouldn't wear certain fragrances in the sun. I'm not sure why, but every once in a while, fragrance plus sun results in an itchy rash. If a mysterious rash develops after a day in the sun, perhaps your perfume caused it. Either change your fragrance, or don't wear it while you're outdoors.

How to Stop Worrying about Your Looks—and Why

I know women, really beautiful women, who dwell on their imperfections. Some of them make themselves miserable worrying about how they're going to improve on—or keep—their looks. They begin to panic at the sight of the first wrinkle. By thirty-five they're already wondering whether it's time yet for a face-lift. Eventually the anxiety begins to show, in the way they talk, in their mannerisms, and most of all in their faces. Someone once said to me, "Don't worry too much

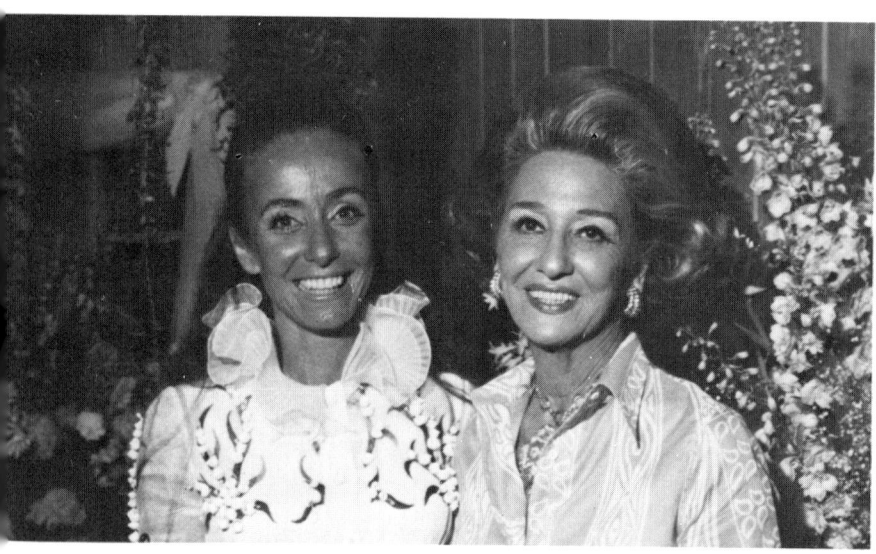

Mothers and daughters: My mother, and my daughter.

(PHOTO: SIDNEY STICKLER)

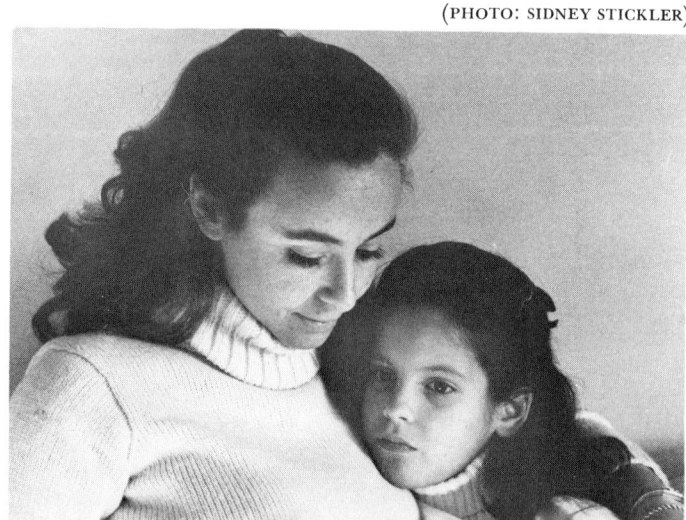

about the way you're going to look three, five, ten years from now because if you do, you're going to end up looking exactly the way you're afraid of looking." I think that person is right.

It's very easy for me or anyone else to dispense advice, to tell you to improve on what can be improved upon—and more important, to accept and not fret about what can't be changed. It may not be so easy for you to follow that advice, especially if you tend to be insecure about your looks. It may involve cultivating a whole new way of seeing and thinking about yourself: instead of you, the would-be great beauty, you can become you, the one-of-a-kind woman with a polished personal style that's yours and yours alone. Think of it that way and all the rest begins to fall into place.

3

Dressing Well

Think of the word "style" and what comes to your mind? To a lot of women—men, too—style means practically the same thing as fashion. (I know. I've tried this little game with some of my friends.)

And why not? We talk about the new styles from Paris and Seventh Avenue. We speak of dressing in the "romantic" style or the "peasant" style. (I'll have more to say about *that* later.)

But we all know that style refers to much more than just fashion. Almost everything is done in a particular style: painting, architecture, literature. There are styles in the way we conduct our day-to-day dealings with other people. And then of course there are styles in cooking, decorating our homes, entertaining, and all the other big and little activities we pursue, which all together make up what we call a life-style.

In the long run, the way a woman dresses is only one aspect of her total style. Still, I happen to believe it's an important aspect. That's because clothes help form our first impression of a person. Whether we like the idea or not, clothes have a lot to do with the way people respond to one another. They can be well or poorly chosen, ultra-conservative or high fashion, flashy, sexy, dowdy, or just plain sloppy; it doesn't matter, they send out powerful messages. Unfortunately, sometimes the messages can be misleading.

Let's imagine a certain woman. She's intelligent and informed, busily absorbed in any number of worthwhile activities. Witty, warm, sympathetic, she's a fascinating conversationalist. Also, a talented organizer, a devoted and loving mother—and good in bed, too. But let's also imagine that this woman often wears uncoordinated, ill-fitting clothes with buttons missing and safety pins holding her skirts closed; that she slops around in rundown shoes; that her coat needs a visit to the cleaner's.

Many of the people she comes into contact with are going to make certain assumptions about her based on what she wears. They're going to get the idea that she's careless, incompetent, not with it; a scatterbrain or worse—that her poor appearance reflects her own low opinion of herself.

Of course, her husband, her children, her good friends and co-workers may know better because they've had the time to get to know her. But what about the people she's just met or the people she thinks she'd enjoy meeting—men and women she'd like to cultivate as friends or as business contacts? Chances are at least some of those other people are going to write her off as a loser.

I don't for one minute believe that dressing well and looking well guarantee success in life, or that simply changing your wardrobe around can help you get ahead on the job (or help advance your husband's career), make you a better wife and mother, revitalize your social life, and enlarge your circle of friends and acquaintances.

My point is simply that clothes communicate, even though they may not say what you want them to say about you. Sloppy, careless dressing makes you appear to be a sloppy, careless person—no matter that you're a meticulous perfectionist in all other areas of your life. In the same way, dressing inappropriately for an event makes it seem as though you either don't know any better, or don't give a damn. And dressing in uniform—wearing exactly what everyone else is wearing that season—makes you seem like an insecure, follow-the-leader type with no initiative or creativity to call your own.

What *about* the way you dress? Do your clothes say what you want them to say about you? Do they reflect the kind of person you really are? The kind of person you want to be?

They can, you know.

In fact, any woman can be well dressed, in a style that communicates her own best image of herself, expresses her individuality, and suits the way she lives. And it doesn't have to cost a king's ransom.

Style vs. Fashion

The woman with "style" isn't necessarily the woman of fashion. In fact, the notion of fashion may be one of the biggest pitfalls of the woman who wants to achieve a unique personal style.

I certainly have nothing against fashion per se. In fact I love it. It's great fun to leaf through the pages of *Vogue* and *Bazaar* and *Women's Wear Daily*. It's marvelous to discover a new fashion look that suits me and the way I live. But I think it's a mistake to take Fashion (note that capital F) too seriously.

When an issue of *Vogue* says, "This is the season for magenta," make a note of it. But for heaven's sake, don't go out and invest heavily in magenta if it's not one of your favorite colors and you don't look well in it. Because as sure as I'm sitting here writing this, one of the next few issues of *Vogue* will come out strongly in favor of some other color. It's the same with everything else that falls under the heading of Fashion. You know it: the "in" thing this season will always be supplanted by next season's "in" thing.

It's not that the people in the fashion business are fickle or trying to put something over on the consumer. Not at all. It's just that the men and women who design, manufacture, and sell fashion are in the business to make money. (And why not? Isn't that what *any* business is all about? And isn't a healthy fashion industry part of a healthy national economy?) But they can't make money unless they can come up with a selection of new fashion looks each season—and create a demand for those new looks.

As for the men and women who edit the fashion publications, their job is to report on those new looks. For the most part, they do a marvelous job. I don't believe for one moment that people like columnist Eugenia Sheppard, Grace Mirabella at *Vogue*, or John Fairchild at *Women's Wear Daily* are trying to con anyone; they're simply keeping people informed of the latest fashion news. It's up to us— you and me and all the other women who read their publications— to decide which of those new fashions we're going to buy and wear.

Unfortunately, too many women confuse style and dressing well with the idea of always being first with the latest fashion looks.

You see this kind of woman practically everywhere, but she's especially visible at fashion shows. I don't go to many fashion shows myself, but when I do get to one, I often find myself paying lots more attention to the show going on in the audience than to the clothes on the runway.

A top-designer fashion show is almost guaranteed to bring out in droves the kind of women I'm tempted to call the "tragedies of fashion." They're a fascinating breed.

Let me give you an example. Last summer I went to a showing of Jimmy Galanos' fall collection. (I have enormous respect for Galanos' designing talents; he and Adolfo are big favorites of mine.) The show was scheduled to start at three in the afternoon. What with shopping and errands, I'd had a busy morning, and because the weather was very hot and muggy, I'd been rushing around town in a linen skirt, sleeveless T-shirt top, sandals, and no stockings. I was running late and rather than go home, change, and put on stockings (it was too hot for them anyway), I dropped my packages off with the doorman and went on to the show. I arrived just as it was about to begin, waved to a few familiar faces, settled down gratefully in the air-conditioned cool, and looked around.

It was 95 degrees outside on that sunny August afternoon, and would you believe that half the women in the audience were dressed for November? Many were wearing boots, sweaters, wool gaucho pants, or heavy midcalf skirts. I even recall seeing at least one fur suit.

Why, you may be wondering, were these otherwise attractive and sensible women wearing fall clothes on a blistering summer day? You can probably guess the answer. Because the clothes they were wearing were not just *any* fall clothes. They were "The New Fall Fashions," probably ordered from other fashion shows held earlier in the season. Each woman was wearing her new purchases in the hope of being *first with the latest.*

Being first with the latest may give some women a great sense of satisfaction. The trouble is, it may also make them look ridiculous. And if there's one thing dressing with style *isn't,* it's ridiculous.

Fashion, as I said before, can be great fun. But the woman who follows fashion blindly, without ever stopping to think about whether this or that look is really right for her, will never be well dressed. Being well dressed starts with using your head. Figuring out who you are. How you want to look. And then choosing your clothes accordingly. It means saying "yes" to some fashions, and an emphatic "no" to others.

Remember 1976 when, for a few months in the fall, something called "the peasant look" was all the rage? It started with Yves St. Laurent's winter collection. The fashion press went gaga. *The New York Times* proclaimed a whole new fashion era. Thousands of women went out and invested (and I do mean *invested;* those clothes were expensive!) in the "rich peasant look"—heavily embroidered tops, longish, full thick skirts, boots, kerchiefs on the head. That kind of thing. On the right woman, under the right circumstances, the look had a certain charm. But one day I saw a family of four filing out of an East Side church with a well-to-do congregation. Daddy came first looking just fine in a conservative business suit. But then came Mommy, Big Sis, and Little Sis, each bundled up in embroidered shawls, fat, gathered skirts, kerchiefs on their heads, and, of course, boots to complete the look. They reminded me of nothing so much as a set of those wooden egg-shaped Ukrainian dolls that you can fit together, one inside the other. All I could think of was "poor, poor peasants."

I wasn't seduced by the peasant look. I live in Manhattan in the last third of the twentieth century. I spend a lot of time rushing around, getting in and out of cabs, making my way down narrow theater aisles, maneuvering between the tables of crowded New York restaurants. I definitely don't live the slow-paced rural life of a nineteenth-century Russian peasant, and the elaborate, voluminous clothing so well suited to that other time and place would be a hindrance to me and the way I live.

I'm aware that it takes a certain amount of courage to ignore a fashion when everyone is grabbing it up. That's a shame, because the woman who aspires to a personal style of her own will never achieve it if she remains a slave to faddish fashions.

Dressing with style means being aware of what's new in fashion and then choosing what's best for you. It means trying gaucho pants (to use just one example), and then rejecting them if they make your rear end look a yard wide and your legs short and stubby.

Women with great style—Babe Paley, for example, and Gloria Guinness and Mirella Agnelli—would *never* wear an unflattering fashion just because someone else (no matter who) says it's "in." And yet, over the years, Paley, Guinness, and Agnelli and a few others continue to be admired for their unique sense of style and fashion savvy. There's a lesson there for any woman who wants to be well dressed.

There *is* a certain relationship between fashion and style, but style always wins out in the long run. So if personal style doesn't mean always being first with the latest, what is it? And how do you get it?

Dress to Please Yourself

My feeling is that a personal style begins with dressing to please yourself—not for the man or men in your life, not to impress other women, but to make *yourself* look and feel attractive.

Many of the women I know claim they dress to please men. Fine. But that means they're making certain assumptions about what men like to see women wear. One woman's version of "dressing to please men" may include wearing clingy fabrics, dresses with deep decolletage, clothes that show a lot of leg. Others assume that men prefer a demure, feminine look—pastel colors, touches of lace, fussy, ruffly blouses instead of tailored shirts. Still others are convinced that the only men worth pleasing prefer women to look "ladylike" and "refined," so they fill their closets with neat shirtwaist dresses, good tweed suits, cashmere sweater sets, and all the other styles symbolic of upper-middle-class suburbia.

They're all dressing to "please men." But men, like women, aren't all pleased by the same things. There's nothing the least bit wrong about adopting any particular "look" as your own. But don't do it as a way of pleasing men. It doesn't work that way.

More important is your *own* feeling about the clothes. No matter how many men it pleases, it's silly to wear a dress with a neckline cut down to the navel if you don't feel comfortable in it. The same goes for ruffly blouses and tweed suits if you don't really like them.

There's another kind of woman who *says* she dresses to please men, but she really dresses to impress women. The fact that she studies *Vogue, Bazaar, Women's Wear Daily,* and the society pages to find out who's wearing what—and then rushes out to buy all the newest looks—is what gives her away.

Let's face it. The subtle ins and outs of women's fashion are lost on the great majority of men. Of course, men want to be proud of their wives, lovers, or dates. (Just as we want to be proud of them.) Of course it makes a man feel good when his female companion looks as though she's chosen her clothes with great care. But unless he's directly involved in the fashion business himself, a man may be totally unaware—and not care in the least—that the shoes you're wearing are all the rage in Paris and the envy of every other woman in the room.

Dressing to impress other women is okay, if that's what makes you happy. But it doesn't help you achieve your goal of developing a unique personal style.

As for dressing to attract or please (or keep) a particular man, it may be worth a try. I know a man who swears he fell in love with his second wife because of what she was wearing the first time he saw her. Their marriage appears to be a good one, but I doubt that it continues to thrive because she dresses to please him. (If dressing to please a mate is all it takes to have a happy marriage, we'd see far fewer divorces.)

I think it's important to listen to the man in your life when he makes suggestions about your clothes. If you always wear crepe and he says he'd love to see you in soft, floaty chiffon, you can at least give chiffon a try—even if it's only in a department store dressing room. Who knows? Chiffon might suit you perfectly. In that case, his suggestion will have helped you define your own personal style.

But if you don't like yourself in chiffon, I'd think twice about buying it. And if your refusal to buy leads to *real* trouble in your relationship, it's pretty safe to assume that the problem between you lies far deeper and is much more serious than disagreement over the clothes you wear.

It's important to make a distinction between dressing to please someone other than yourself and learning from someone who knows what they're talking about.

I learned a lot from Norman Norell. Yes, he's dead now (and I miss him). And yes, fashions have changed since then. But some things, the basic principles, never change. I learned some of those basic principles from him—more about that is coming up—but all the time he encouraged me to modify what I learned to suit myself, to make my own decisions. In short, to dress to please myself.

How to Have "Clothes Sense"

It's easy for me to advise you to start wearing what makes you happy. But I also know that some women (perhaps you're one of them?) haven't the faintest idea where or how to begin. This may be because

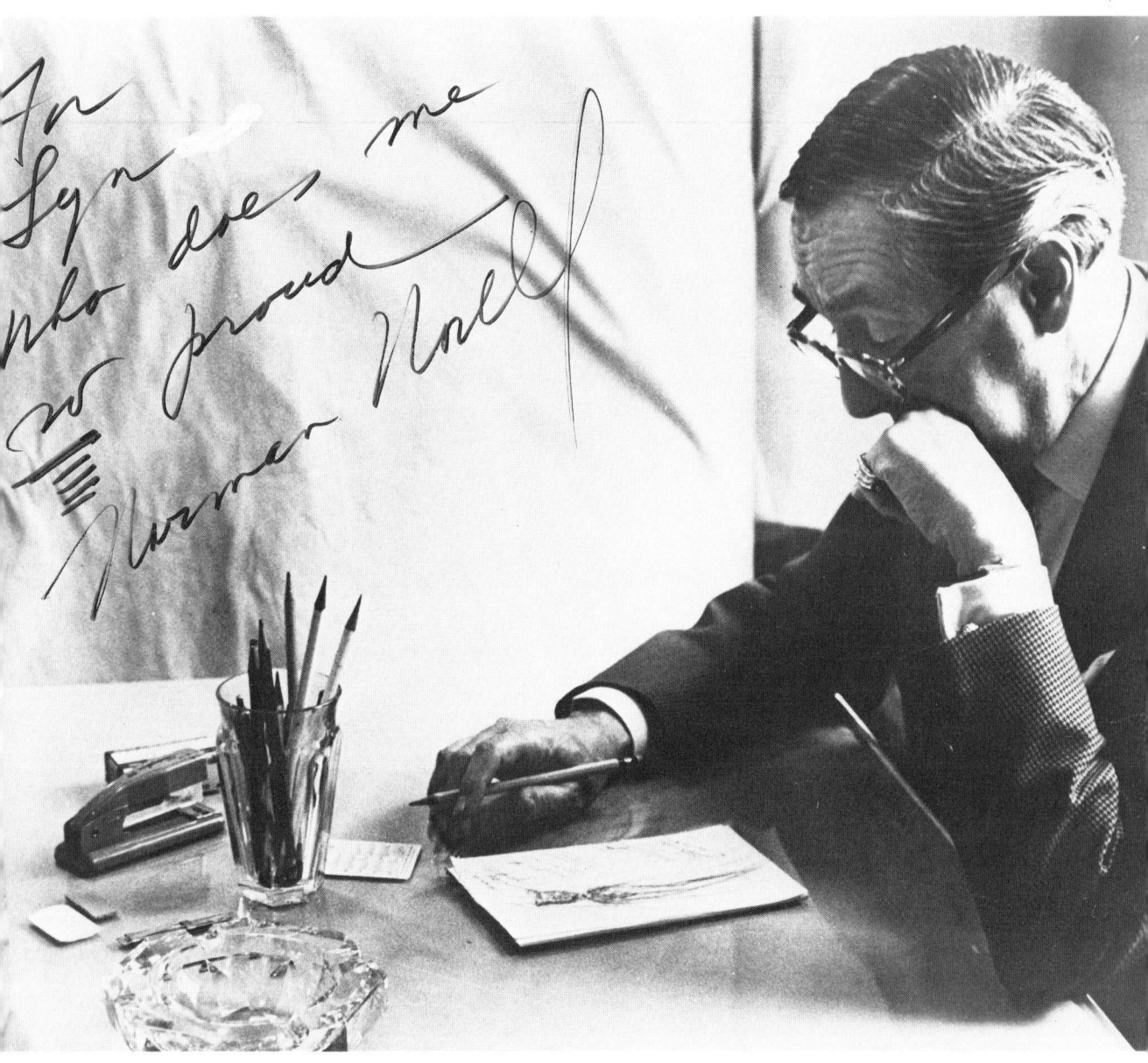

Norman Norell, a personal friend and the dean of American fashion designers.

NORMAN NORELL INCORPORATED   *Friday*

Dear Lynn

I had such a good time last night — I'm "not much for those things" but I *did* have a great time. I realized last night that all the compliments last night on the dress were *really* for you, Lynn, — (you would have to be a really *rotten* designer to make you look anything less than marvelous)

Thanks again
& love
Norman

550 SEVENTH AVENUE, NEW YORK, NEW YORK 10018   CHICKERING 4-5452

---

n d n

Dear Lyn:

I had such a good time Wednesday evening. I did enjoy the ballet and going to El Morocco was a treat for me — I go out so seldom — It was fun to see the "get ups" on people — they sure do "get a 'rarely'" there. Thanks again

Norman

Norell wrote very few personal letters. That's why I treasure these so much.

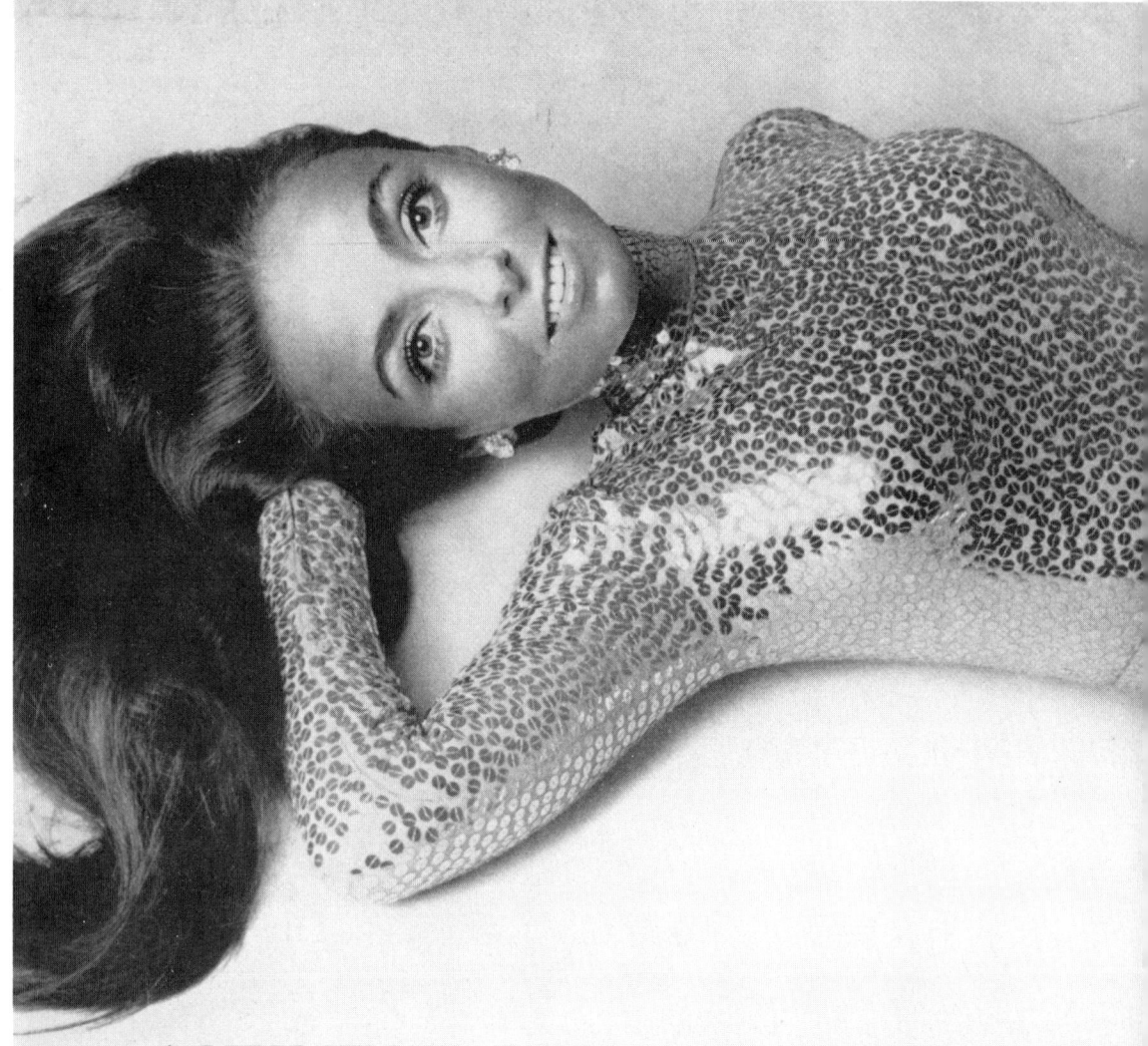

A NUMBER ONE FAN
Lyn Revson in the newest Norells

Lyn, Mrs. Charles Revson, a petite brunette with spectacular eyes and a ditto figure, has been a Norman Norell fan since she bought her first one at age eighteen. Since then, the Revson N. N. collection has grown to "about fifty things that I wear constantly—and about one hundred more that are put away—for the moment." The fact that Mrs. Revson has never discarded a single Norell—just keeps rotating them in and out of her current life—says a lot about a Norell. It means they are clothes that work for a modern woman who demands and needs a lot of things simultaneously from her wardrobe— glamour, beautiful color, newness of line, superb fabrics; but also timelessness, classic simple shapes and a comfortable practicality that can take her around a fast-moving life. Say, after three weeks at sea on the Revson yacht, the Ultima II, the Revsons, on a moment's notice, drop in for a gala dinner in Monte Carlo. Lyn is sensational in sizzling sequins. It seems that a Norell sequin dress folds flat as a sweater on a shelf. Here, three of the great new Norell looks that combine everything he stands for—all the elements that make for true luxury: glamour, elegance, longevity, and practicality....

"A Number One Fan: Lyn Revson in the newest Norells..." That's what they said in thi

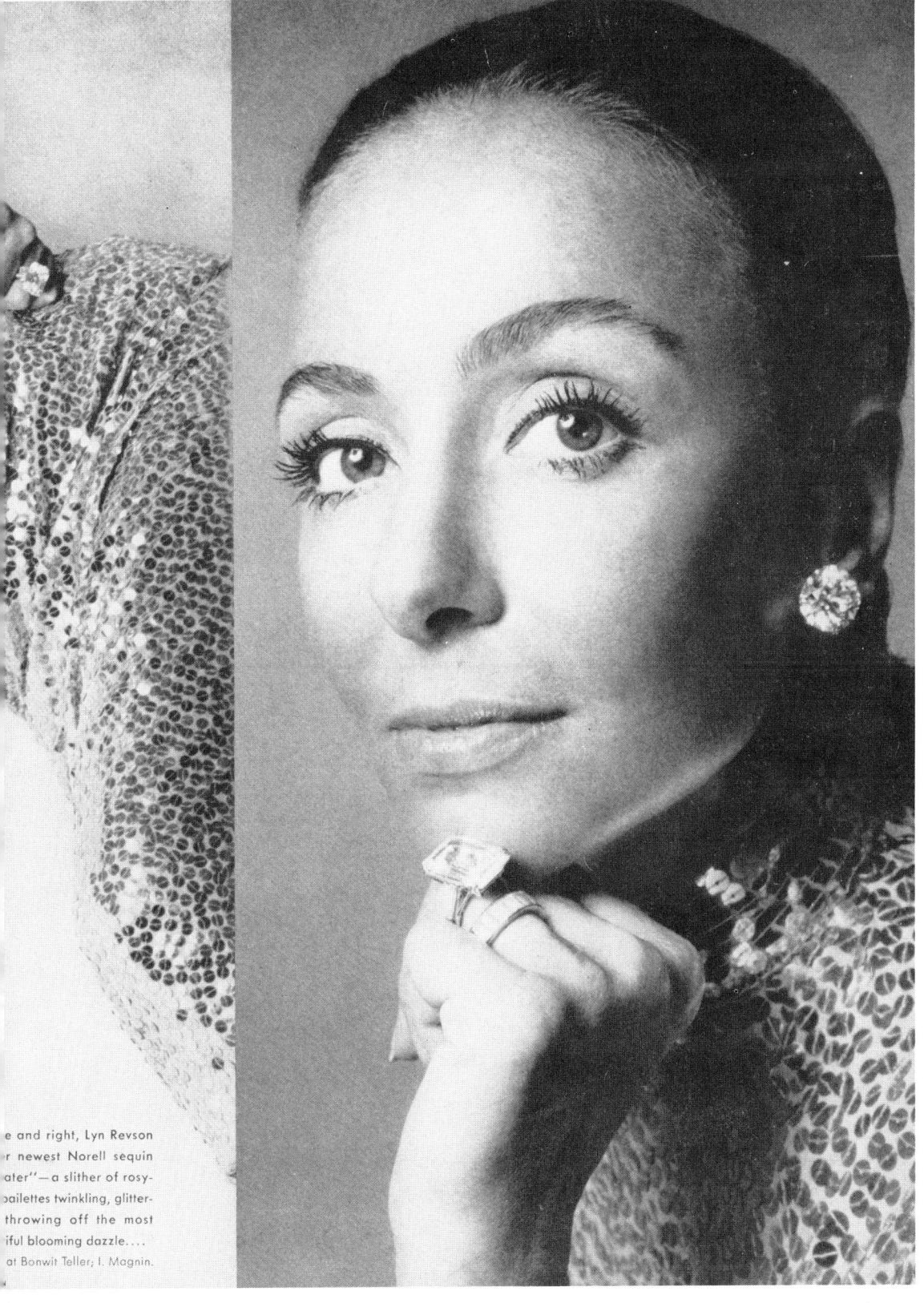

e and right, Lyn Revson
 newest Norell sequin
ater"—a slither of rosy-
ailettes twinkling, glitter-
throwing off the most
iful blooming dazzle....
at Bonwit Teller; I. Magnin.

ayout which appeared in a 1973 issue of *Vogue*.

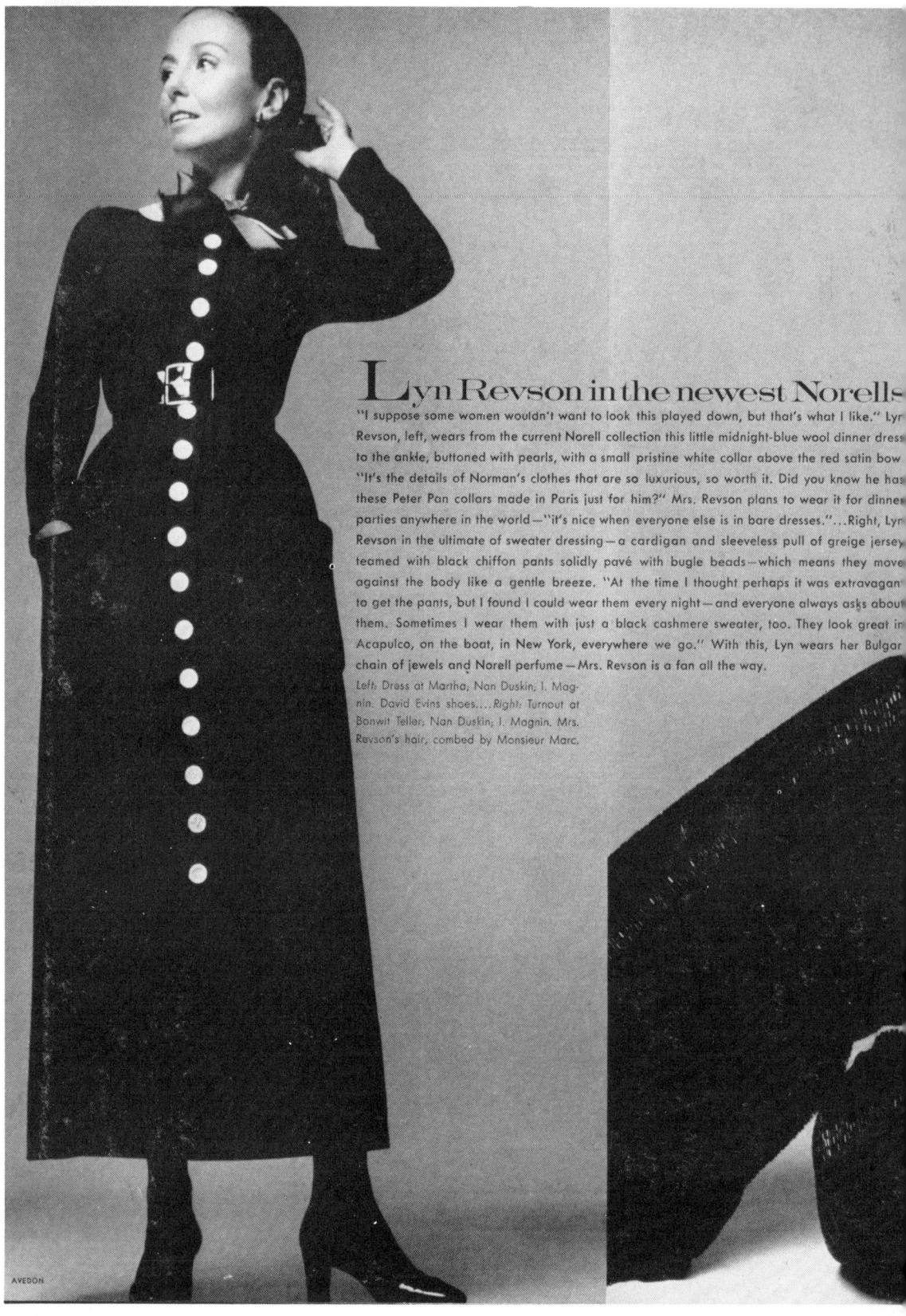

Lyn Revson in the newest Norells

"I suppose some women wouldn't want to look this played down, but that's what I like." Lyn Revson, left, wears from the current Norell collection this little midnight-blue wool dinner dress to the ankle, buttoned with pearls, with a small pristine white collar above the red satin bow. "It's the details of Norman's clothes that are so luxurious, so worth it. Did you know he has these Peter Pan collars made in Paris just for him?" Mrs. Revson plans to wear it for dinner parties anywhere in the world—"it's nice when everyone else is in bare dresses."...Right, Lyn Revson in the ultimate of sweater dressing—a cardigan and sleeveless pull of greige jersey, teamed with black chiffon pants solidly pavé with bugle beads—which means they move against the body like a gentle breeze. "At the time I thought perhaps it was extravagant to get the pants, but I found I could wear them every night—and everyone always asks about them. Sometimes I wear them with just a black cashmere sweater, too. They look great in Acapulco, on the boat, in New York, everywhere we go." With this, Lyn wears her Bulgari chain of jewels and Norell perfume—Mrs. Revson is a fan all the way.

Left: Dress at Martha, Nan Duskin, I. Magnin. David Evins shoes....Right: Turnout at Bonwit Teller, Nan Duskin, I. Magnin. Mrs. Revson's hair, combed by Monsieur Marc.

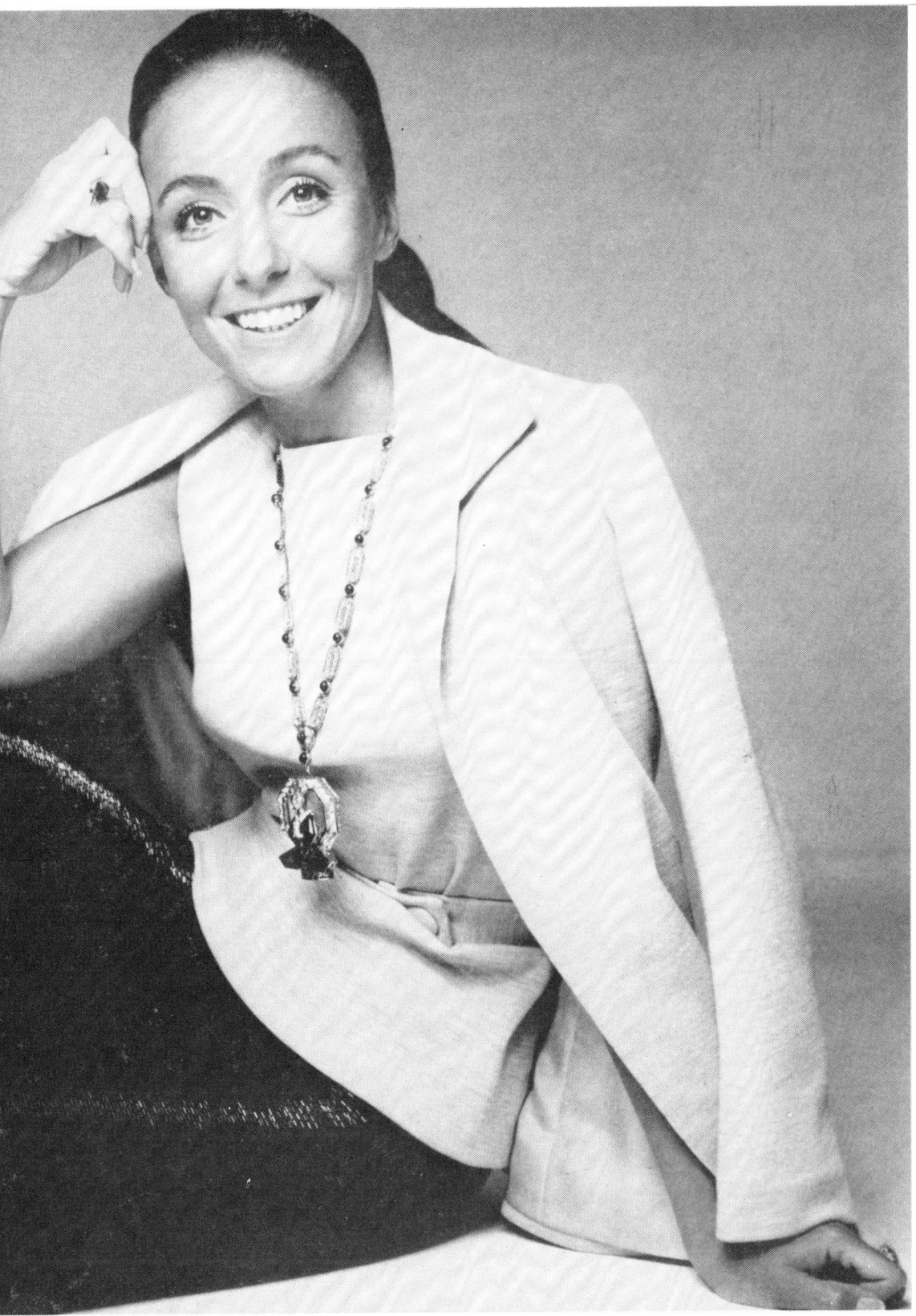

you've been following fashion all your life and never had the chance to develop a clothes sense of your own. Or it may be because you've always dressed with the idea of impressing or pleasing someone else. No matter. You *can* have clothes sense if you're willing to put a little time and effort into it.

First you have to have taste. It's impossible to define "good" taste and "bad" taste; everyone's version is different. That's okay; the idea is to develop your *own* taste. For this, you need exposure. If you're unsure of your own taste, start looking at the fashion magazines. Spend time at some of the better stores in your area, absorbing the look and feel of beautifully made clothes. Study the way other women put themselves together, especially the ones who've gotten a reputation for their own clothes sense. Be critical. Decide which looks appeal to you, which don't, and try to figure out why. Learn the rules so that you'll be able to break them if you want to.

This process, easy to describe in just a few words, may take a little while to come together in your own head. I can't predict how long, but little by little, your own sense of taste will become sharper, more acute.

Soon you'll be ready to apply what you've learned to yourself.

To begin you have to give some thought to your physical assets. These, of course, you want to emphasize. Your defects, or shortcomings, should be minimized.

Let me give you a few examples of what I mean. My legs are pretty good. So for years now, I've been wearing my skirts at a precise nineteen inches from the floor, which means they stop just at the middle of the knee. When other women were wearing their skirts much shorter, some of my well-meaning friends in the fashion business were after me to have my hems taken up. But I don't like bare knees for city dressing (tennis clothes and casual skirts and dresses for the country are something else again). So, I kept my skirts at mid-knee length.

Now that fashion decrees the somewhat longer skirt, these same well-meaning friends tell me I ought to lengthen mine. But I know what I like and don't like and I feel midcalf-length skirts are unattractive. And besides, why cover up one of my best features—my legs?

So my reply to their kindly (I assume) criticisms is always a "Thank you, but I feel best in a knee-length skirt." Despite the fact that for years I haven't gone along with the ups and downs of hemlines, I've been on the Best-Dressed List four times and have a permanent place in the Fashion Hall of Fame.

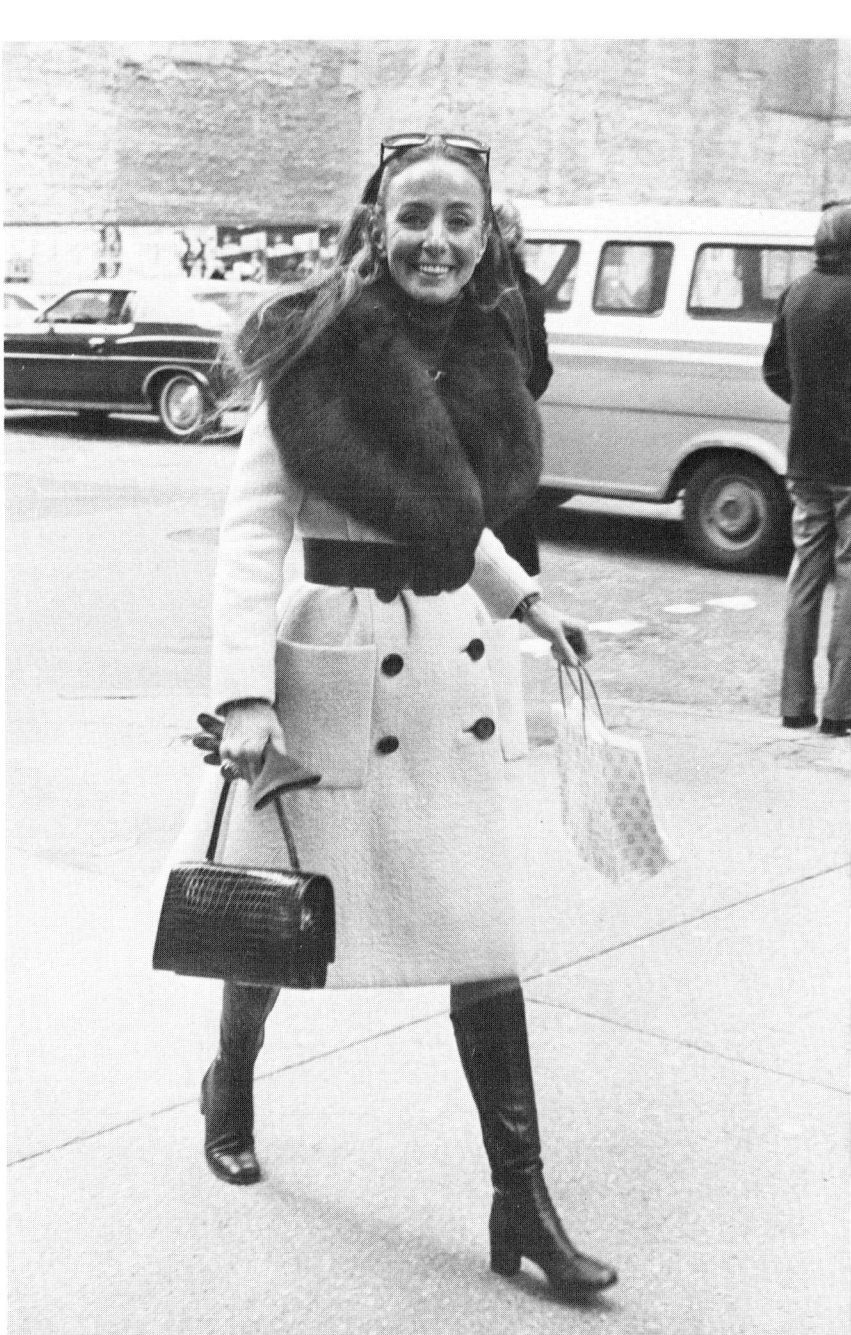

Women's Wear Daily says this nine-year-old Norell coat is too short, but regardless of fashion, knee-length coats and skirts are my best look. (PHOTO: NICK MACHALABA/WWD)

Another example: I have a small waist. I consider that an asset, too. In general, I prefer clothes that define my waist and avoid dresses, smock tops, or anything else that ignores the waistline. But I'm long-waisted and short from waist to crotch. That's not exactly a defect, but it does present certain problems. It means that unless I want to have my pants custom-made I have to seek out and choose the kind that have no waistband and which ride rather low on the hips. (The waistband on most ready-made pants hits me somewhere around the middle of the rib cage!)

A final example: because of the size of my chest, the blouson style is not a good one on me. Those dresses with the generously cut bloused tops that many designers are showing in their latest collections make me look like a nursing mother! So I avoid that style completely.

As you can see, I'm aware of my body and how certain styles flatter or detract from it. Your good (and not so good) points may be—and probably are—quite different from mine. It doesn't matter. Get to know your own body type. Stand in front of a mirror and try to be objective about what you see. Both the good and the bad. No one's perfect. But each of us has physical features that are attractive—maybe even sensational. And the less attractive aspects of our bodies? Some can be changed. You can lose weight if need be, firm up certain areas, even resort to plastic surgery if you feel you must. But some things you're stuck with. (A short neck, for example, or unusually broad shoulders.) Own up to these flaws and always keep them in mind when you start selecting new clothes for your wardrobe.

There's more to developing clothes sense than simply learning to choose clothes that flatter the outer, physical you. If your style is going to be personal, a reflection of you (and no other style matters), it must also express your *feelings* about yourself and the image of the inner you that you want to communicate to others.

For example, I see myself as an honest, straightforward person. I don't play games or beat around the bush. (In fact, it's been suggested to me more than once that I cultivate the habit of thinking first and speaking later.) I'm not devious, or coy, or complicated. What I am is what I appear to be. A direct, natural, uncomplicated look goes along with my personality. Just as I'm not a gimmicky person, I don't like gimmicky clothes. Just as I don't change my opinions or loyalties from month to month, I also tend to maintain certain constants in my wardrobe.

You may be very different. Perhaps more complex and introspective. You may be drawn to the romantic—possibly even the exotic or bizarre. My classic, straightforward way of dressing could be all wrong for you because it wouldn't reflect the subtleties of your personality. You might be happier instead in clothes with a touch of mystery, intrigue.

Or, you might see yourself as the ultimate sensuous woman (or at least want to get that message across to some of the important people in your life). In that case you'd want to communicate some of your earthy warmth, perhaps by wearing rich, deep colors, fabrics that are inviting to the touch.

Or again you might be outgoing, gregarious, exuberant. A take-charge personality, always happiest in the limelight—or at least backstage directing the show. Clothes that attract attention, in bright colors, with dramatic lines, might suit you best.

I can't possibly know the physical characteristics of each woman who reads this book, much less the inner ones that make her unique. But I don't need to. Once you begin to know yourself, outside and in, you're on your way to developing "clothes sense" and a distinctive style all your own.

Fashion Mistakes and How to Learn from Them

Even women with clothes sense make an occasional mistake; you'll find one or two accidents in almost everyone's closet. It's a shame to waste money on clothes that are hardly ever worn, but there's a brighter side to the picture: you can *learn* from your mistakes.

Let me tell you about a recent mistake of mine.

I'm what you might call an "instinctive" shopper. (Though maybe it's not instinct at all; maybe I understand myself well enough by now so I don't have to stop and figure out whether I like something or not. I just know.) In any event, I tend to go by first impressions of a dress, or shirt, or scarf, or whatever, and I've learned that if an article of clothing (or a piece of jewelry or furniture, or even a person, for that matter) doesn't appeal to me immediately, it probably never will.

So not too long ago I was in Jax on Fifty-seventh Street. I've been shopping there for twenty-five years. I came across a very simple basic black cotton knit dress, the kind that's cut like a T-shirt. Now, T-shirt dresses are smart and practical and I knew I'd be needing a couple of new ones for the summer. But there was an indefinable "something" about this one that didn't hit me just right.

I tried it on anyway and studied it, and me, in the mirror. Nothing to get excited about. There was none of that thrill of recognition—that feeling of "this is really me"—that I always look for when I buy something new. In fact, it was a rather "blah" dress. But there was nothing really *wrong* with it either. Finally I said to myself, "Why not? With a bright scarf at the neckline and an attractive belt, I might get some wear out of it." So I bought the dress.

Well, do you know what? I haven't worn it once. When indeed would I *want* to wear it? I certainly don't want to wear a "blah" dress when *I'm* feeling "blah." On those days, I want something that picks me up and makes me feel better. I don't want to wear a "blah" dress when I'm feeling good either. The dress would bring me down.

I have nothing against basic black dresses. I have a couple and when I wear them I feel marvelous. The point of the story is this: my clothes sense—my instincts, if you want to call it that—told me this wasn't the dress for me. But, carried away by the idea of "practicality," I bought it anyway. It'll be a long time before I make that kind of mistake again. (Incidentally, the story has a happy ending. My daughter Susan saw the dress in my closet, tried it on, and looked sensational! It's hers now.)

A lot of fashion mistakes are made because the woman allows the idea of "practicality," or Fashion, or someone else's opinion of what she ought to wear override her own clothes sense.

If your clothes sense isn't yet fully developed, you can help it along by studying some of the mistakes already hanging in your closet. Haul them out, try them on, and take a good long look at yourself in each one. Try to analyze what it is you don't like about each one.

Is it too safe? Boring? Did you buy it only because it was practical? Practical clothes should be simple, but they don't have to be dull. Next time, look for something with a little more zip. And remember, though you may never learn to really love a dull little dress, you may start wearing it more often if you can find ways to liven it up with a scarf, belt, chains, etc.

Is the dress too "far out" in terms of line, cut, design? Did you buy it because at the time it seemed like the very last word in capital F Fashion? Well, there's another lesson. Fashion extremes may be fun to wear for a while, but they do become obsolete almost overnight. Nobody wants to walk around in a dress that practically screams out the year and season it was "born." I make it my policy never to buy fashion fads—never, in other words, to invest in a look that is so "of the moment" that no one had even dreamed of anything like it the year before. (In fact, my favorite clothes are the ones that go on and on. I have dresses, skirts, and suits in my closets that date back twelve years and more. They're timeless. I still wear them and I still love them.)

Next time you go out to buy a dress, keep in mind that if it's startlingly new the season you buy it, it's going to be hopelessly dated by the next season. There's not much you can do with an outdated fashion fad except to give it away, or pack it away in a trunk and hope the fad is revived in your lifetime.

Is there something about the way the dress is made that bothers you? I'm not referring to *fit* here, but to things like the shape of the neckline; the fabric; whether it's high-waisted, low-waisted, or no-waisted; has set-in sleeves or raglan sleeves; a full skirt or a very narrow one. If you know that you don't like a particular dress because it has a high waistline or raglan sleeves, you're going to be extra careful about buying anything else with a high waistline or raglan sleeves. Result: fewer fashion mistakes in the future.

While you're going over past mistakes, you might also want to take another look at some of the success stories in your closet. Almost every woman owns at least one or two outfits that do marvelous things for her. Again, try to figure out what makes those particular clothes such fun to wear. Does it have to do with color? Fabric? Shape? The details of the way they're made? Perhaps it's a combination of things. Whatever, look for more of the same when you're shopping for new clothes.

Obviously, I'm not suggesting that you go out and buy four more lime-green linen dresses because you once had a lime-green linen dress that you adored. Or that you should never again consider a rust-colored skirt if you once had one that you hated. There's nothing to be gained by being *that* rigid. But you *can* be guided in a basic, general way by your past mistakes—and successes.

How to Build a Wardrobe

Whether you're happy with the clothes you have or not, I think I can safely assume that you have a closetful of them. Most women do.

But there's a big difference between owning a closetful of clothes and having a wardrobe that works in dozens of different ways and takes you almost anywhere. With a random closetful of clothes, even if most of them are clothes you like, you can still end up in one of those frustrating situations where you've got someplace to go but nothing quite right to wear. With a good wardrobe that can't happen.

The basic ideas behind the wardrobe I'm going to tell you how to build come from none other than the great Norman Norell, perhaps the most talented designer America has ever produced, and a man who cared enormously not only about clothes but about women and how we want to look. His suggestions were invaluable to me, and it gives me great pleasure to be able to pass them on to you.

Before I do, let me assure you I'm not recommending that you scrap everything you already own and start fresh with the guidelines given here. Instead, keep what you have and gradually add to your own collection of clothes until you've accumulated all the basics on the list. (You may already have some of those basics. So much the better.)

To begin, let's think of winter, first. Norell once told me that a woman can't go wrong if she starts out with a black skirt and white blouse. (However, if you've got a great pants figure, or simply feel more comfortable in pants, you might want to modify Norell's advice and make a pair of beautifully fitting black pants the backbone of your wardrobe.)

If you go with the skirt, look for one in lightweight wool. It should have "easy" lines and be neither *too* full nor pencil slim. As for the blouse, it should be silk and tailored—no ruffles, please, and no big balloon sleeves—but it needn't be severe. Instead of stark snowy white, consider a soft, slightly creamy white, which is more flattering to most complexions and more versatile in terms of the colors you can team it with.

How much should you pay for your skirt and blouse? Since they may be the two most important items in your wardrobe, it will be worth it in the long run to spend as much as you need to—or as much as you can—for good quality, fabric, and workmanship. That doesn't mean they have to come from a name designer; it does mean that they should be well made and not obviously from the bargain basement. (It's possible, though, that with a keen eye and a highly developed knack for locating "good buys," you could find good fabric, cut, and fit—in short, just what you're looking for—in a bargain basement.)

This is a good rule for *anything* you buy: *always* look for the best quality—the best fabric and workmanship—at the price you can afford.

Now let's consider what you can do with that black skirt and white blouse. For a sporty look, buckle a good leather belt around your waist, add tights or textured stockings, and boots or medium-heeled shoes. Another way to vary the look for day wear would be to loop a long, rectangular scarf under the collar of the blouse and tie it loosely in front so that the ends float free.

At night, you can wear the blouse with the first two or three buttons undone, fill in the neckline with gold (or gold-look) chains, or a strand of pearls. Wear gold or pearl earrings, switch to sheer stockings and strippy high-heeled shoes, and you have a "little evening" look that's perfect for the theater, restaurants, movies, and informal evenings at someone's house.

(I practically "lived" in this evening look all during the winter of 1976, when everyone else was wearing peasant clothes and midcalf skirts with boots. More precisely, I bought myself two Mila Schön skirts, one white, one black, and three silk shirts: white, pink, and navy. I wore the skirts and shirts in various combinations, dressed them up with chains or pearls, sometimes tied a scarf around my waist instead of a belt. I always felt perfectly well dressed and even though 1977 brought clothes that I like better than the ones everyone wore in 1976, I'll always be a firm believer in the right shirt and skirt for evening. It's always a marvelous look, a classic, and I'll continue to wear it.)

Once you've got the black skirt and white silk shirt, your next purchase probably should be a V-neck or turtleneck sweater. Again, buy a good one: wool or cashmere, if you can afford it. And have it in a color that you won't tire of easily.

This last bit of advice is very important if you don't own a lot of clothes. Red might be your favorite color, but if your wardrobe is small you might be wearing that red sweater several times a week. Do you love red *that* much?

Norell's advice was to start out with the neutrals: black and white, followed by beige and gray. They all work beautifully together, and you don't get tired of them easily.

Back to the sweater. Wear it alone with the black skirt. Or layer it under (if it's a turtleneck) or over (if it's a V-neck) the white silk blouse. The result is another great daytime look, perfect for work, or for shopping or lunches.

Item number 4 would be a gray flannel skirt, possibly pleated (but only if you look good in pleats) or slightly gathered at the waistline. Charcoal gray is best.

The gray flannel skirt, with the white blouse or sweater, or both, gives you a daytime look that's a little less dressed up, more casual, than the black skirt.

After that, more tops. Perhaps a black silk blouse (wear it with the black skirt and you have an instant basic black "dress" to accessorize up or down), and another wool or cashmere sweater (one with a "standard" round sweater neckline). Finally, a third sweater for dressier evenings. I have a black one with metallic threads running through it, and when I wear it with a black skirt I feel very dressed up indeed. The look is appropriate for almost any evening event except for formal ones, which call for a long gown.

What else goes into a basic wardrobe?

Well, to begin with, a pair of superbly fitting jeans. Obviously, hardly anyone today can get by without them. (I practically live in mine and one of my very favorite looks consists of jeans, a cashmere sweater, and an extravagant piece of real jewelry—a giant emerald or ruby ring, for example.)

A jacket or blazer, preferably one with a sleek fit through the waist and shoulders, like a riding jacket. Especially useful in a fabric like velveteen or corduroy (soft, buttery suede might be good, too), you can toss this kind of jacket over almost anything to achieve a smart, pulled-together look. Try to find one in a color you can team with the other basics in your wardrobe. Garnet might be a good choice. Or chocolate brown.

A winter coat. Fur if you can manage it, since fur can take you just about anywhere these days, from the supermarket to opening nights at the opera. If not fur, then good-quality wool in a neutral color, a classic nongimmicky style.

A slicker, poncho, or trench coat to wear in the rain.

A pair of brown leather medium-heeled walking shoes.

A pair of beige or black high-heeled shoes.

A pair of sneakers. (I buy mine at Indian Walk, the children's shoe store.)

Rubber rain boots.

A good leather shoulder bag for day. (A top-quality bag can be one of your best investments. I have bags that are twenty years old and they keep getting better and better with time.)

An evening bag. (Metallic gold or silver bags have been very popular for a while now; everyone seems to want one. I prefer fabric.

There's less chance of someone coming along and walking away with it. The truth is, I often end up not carrying any bag at night. The only thing I really need is a compact, and that I can slip into my pocket.)

A medium-width dark brown or black leather belt. (But don't forget the trick of adding color and unexpected chic by wrapping and tying a vivid-colored scarf at your waist.)

For color, scarves in all shapes and sizes. (Plus, if you can afford it, a large beige or ivory-colored shawl that can be layered and tied any-which-way over practically anything else in the wardrobe. Not necessarily a "basic," but certainly nice to have for its added warmth and drama.)

Chains. Real gold or gold-look.

Gloves for the cold. Fur-lined gloves are nice, but you can get

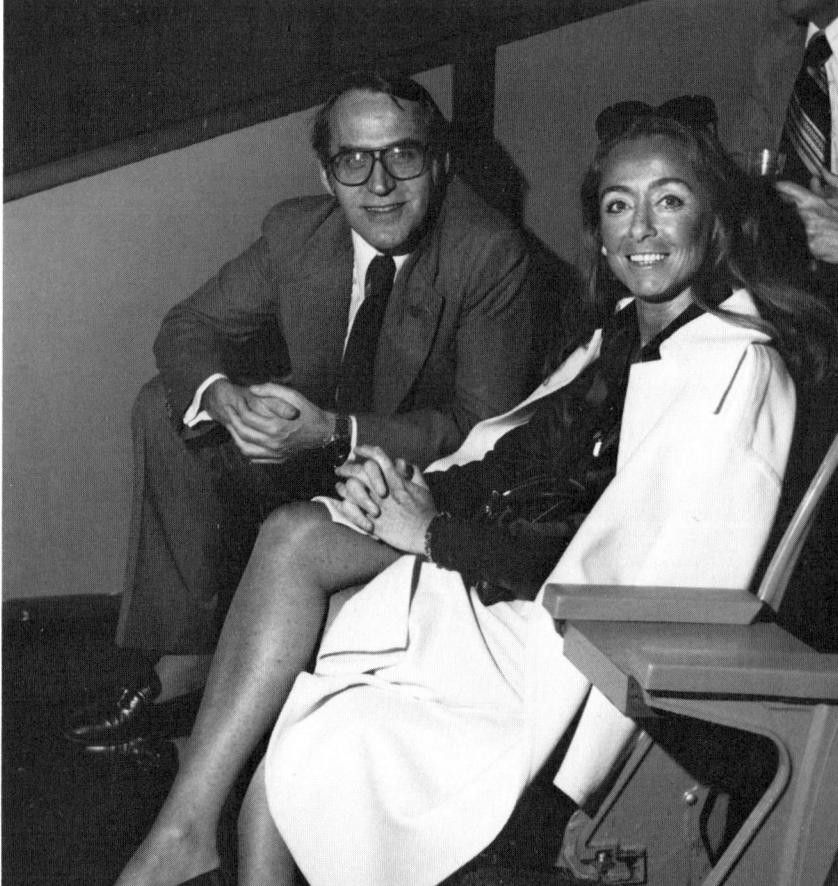

A silk shirt and wool skirt go practically anywhere. Here at a baseball game with New York City Commissioner of Cultural Events, Neil Walsh, I'm wearing Jimmy Galanos' vanilla-colored skirt with coat to match.

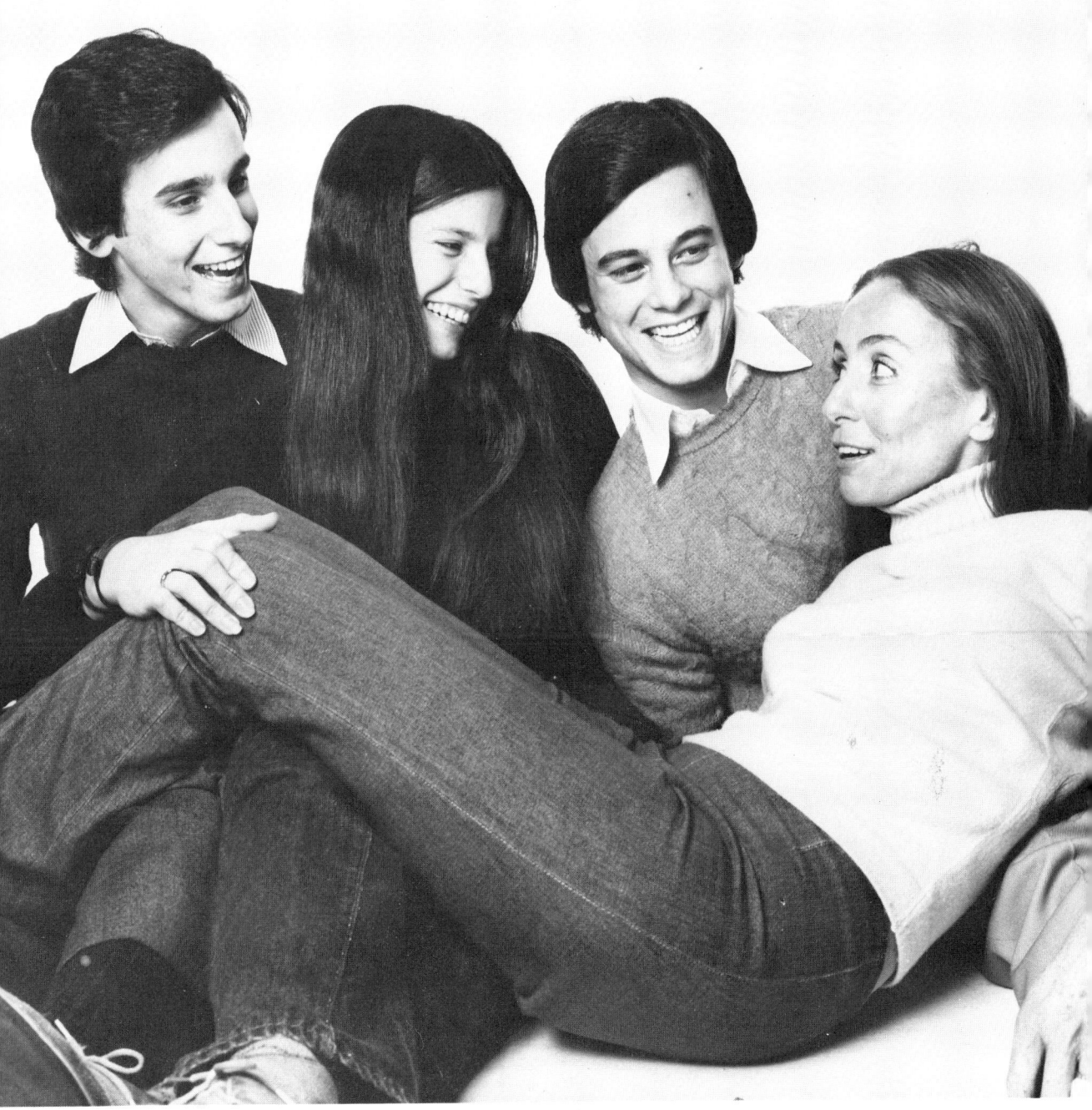

Turtleneck sweater and jeans: one of my favorite looks, worn here with three of my favorite people—my children Jeffrey, Susan, and Steven.

lovely, soft cashmere gloves in white or beige for about $8.95 at Bloomingdale's and other stores.

You may be wondering whatever happened to the street-length dress and why I haven't mentioned it till now. As you've probably guessed, my personal preference is for separates. But that isn't the main reason for not emphasizing dresses. I've focused on separates because two or three tops and a couple of skirts can take you more places, give you a wider variety of different looks, than two or three dresses can—and usually for less money, too.

My advice is not to give too much thought to dresses until you've collected a small wardrobe of separates. *Then* add a dress or two.

As for which kind, of course be guided by what looks best on you. However, it's my feeling that the simple knit dress, cut like a long T-shirt, is the most versatile and useful of all. (If you're going to have two, get one in a dark color and one in a light shade.)

Those are the basics that will see you through any occasion, with the exception of a formal dinner or ball. For that, you'll need a long dress or skirt and top, the more spectacular the better.

Now for summer: if anything, a basic summer wardrobe is even easier to put together than one for cooler weather.

To begin with, you've already got jeans, right? Add a pair of white cotton duck pants for day (I've been getting marvelous white duck pants at Jax for years) and white crepe pants for evening. Then get two or three cotton T-shirts to team with the jeans and white duck pants. You can wear the silk shirts from your winter wardrobe with the white crepe pants for a dressed-up "little evening" look.

Finally, two cotton or silk knit T-shirt dresses, one short, in a light color, for day, the other dark, and perhaps long, for evening.

The same scarves, chains, and belts you use to accessorize a winter wardrobe can be used to dress your summer clothes up or down.

You'll also need a bathing suit. (And a tennis dress if that's your sport.)

A big straw bag.

A pair of sandals in beige or bone leather. (Silk espadrilles would be nice, too.)

And that just about does it for the basics.

Another favorite look of mine: the hacking jacket (this from Knoud's, a Madison Avenue riding store), turtleneck sweater, beautifully tailored pants from Hermès. (PHOTO: NICK MACHALABA/WWD)

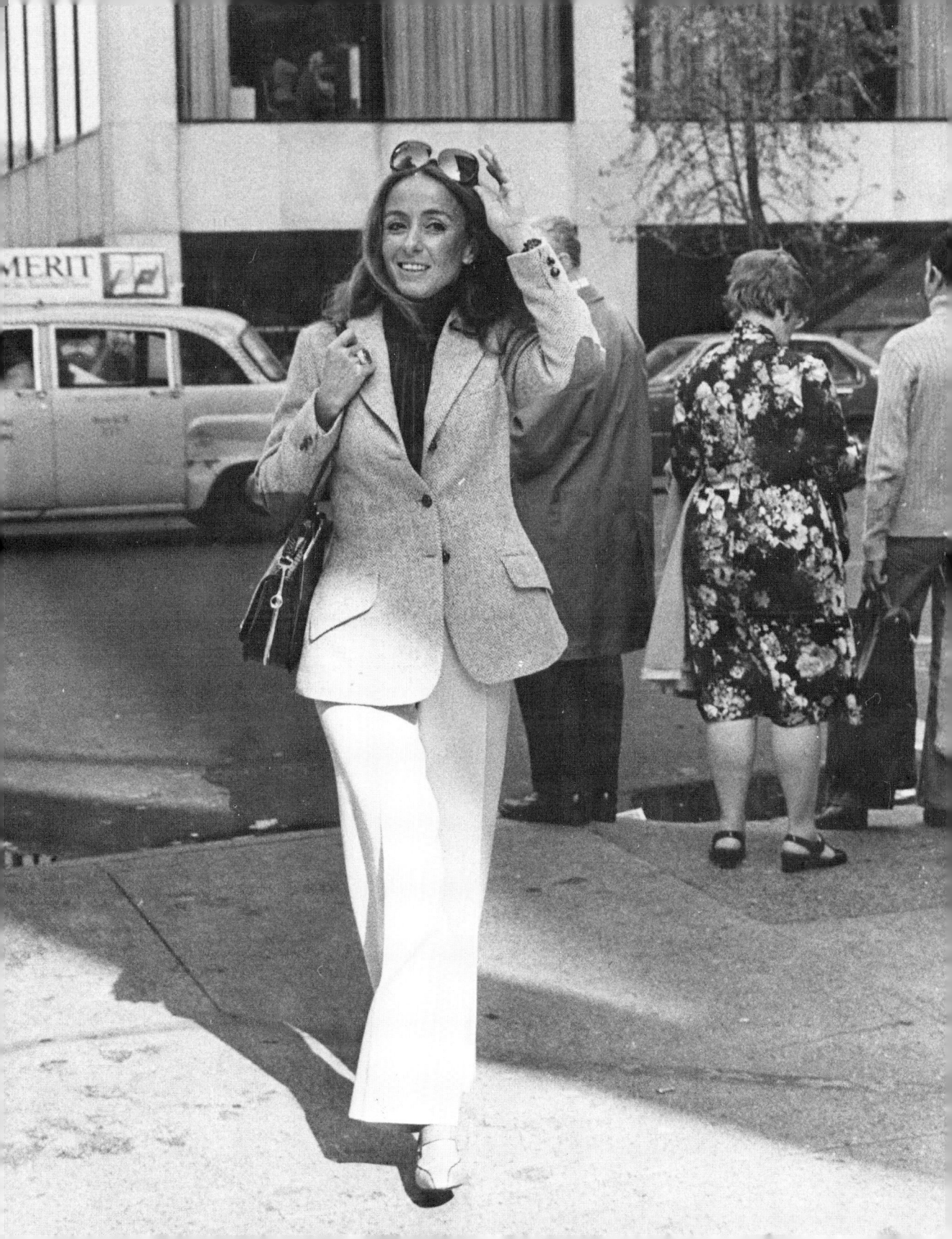

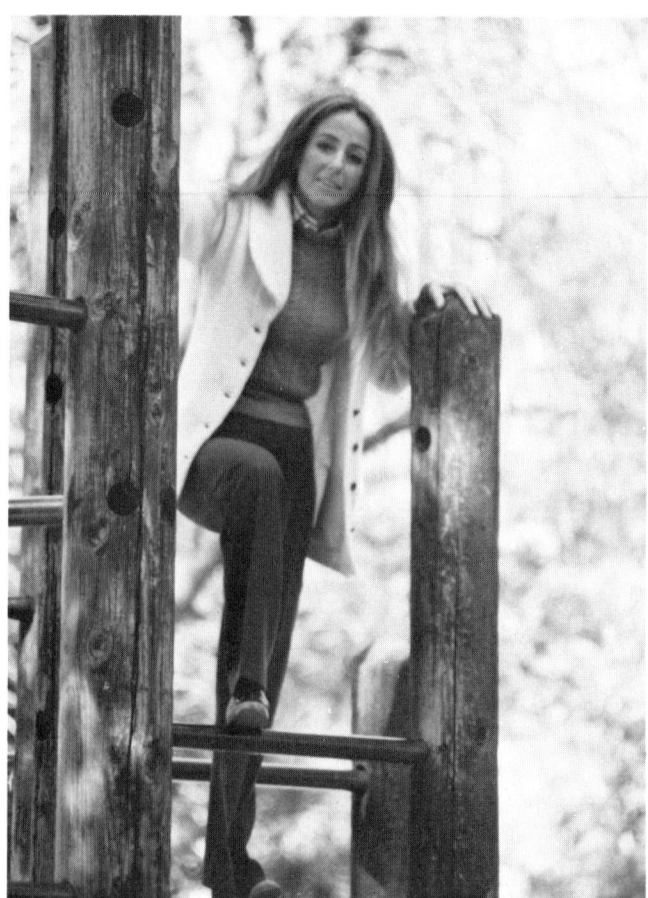

Gray flannel pants (these are from Hermès), a shirt, and layers of sweaters—just the thing for Saturday in Central Park, or any park. (PHOTO: LEE GUBER)

In Venice with Bern and Billy Rose. Cream-white silk shirt and lightest weight cream wool pants (from Hermès) are great for travel. So's the roomy Hermès bag.

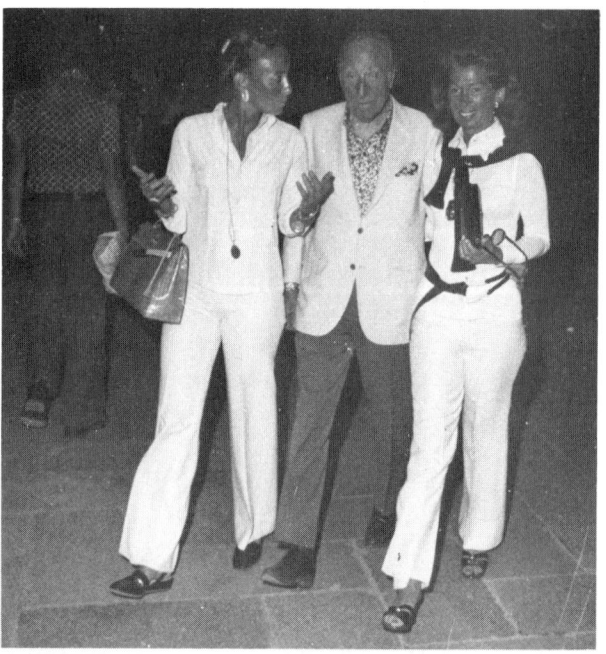

A Few Dos and Don'ts for Building a Wardrobe

You don't need to have a lot of clothes or a lot of money to be well dressed. Not if you have a small "core" collection of separates that work together in many different ways to give you a variety of different looks. That's what the basic wardrobe I've just outlined does.

Throughout, I've emphasized neutral colors because black, grays, whites, creams, ivories, and beiges can be teamed in practically any combination and still look rich and "pulled together." But unless those neutrals are your favorite colors to begin with (as they are for me), at some point you're going to want to add more color and pattern to your clothes.

That's where your own individuality enters the picture. That's also where a lot of women start making some major mistakes. Not trusting their own color sense, overly influenced by the fashion magazines and beauty books, their friends, the men in their lives, they start adding color every which way. The result is a hodgepodge—blouses, skirts, sweaters, and dresses in a rainbow of hues that may be lovely to look at hanging there in a closet but severely cut back on the versatility of a wardrobe.

You don't have to commit yourself to certain colors for life. It's only natural for color preferences to change somewhat over the years. But if you want a coordinated wardrobe, you are going to have to start making certain decisions about color. And stick to them, at least for a while.

How do you make those decisions? Simple. Think of the colors you like best, the ones you find yourself reaching for whenever all else is equal and you have a choice. Are they the bright sunny reds, oranges, and yellows? The delicate pastels? Deep jewel tones such as garnet, sapphire, emerald? Are they the sophisticated grayed shades—teal blues, dusty roses, maroons? Earthy colors like pumpkin, brown, plum? Chances are, whatever your favorite colors in general, they'll be the ones you'll most enjoy wearing. It would be a good idea to concentrate on them—instead of going off on wild tangents—when adding color to your wardrobe.

But what if you think you don't look well in your favorite colors? What if you read in a magazine or beauty book that, based on your complexion and hair, your favorite colors are the very ones you should avoid wearing?

I think you can guess how I feel about that. It's all nonsense. You're much better off wearing a particular color because you love it than wearing a color you loathe because some beauty or fashion expert says you should.

Of course, some colors *are* more flattering to some women than others. But most women can wear any color they like. If you're mad for a particular color but *you* feel it doesn't look well on you, try to figure out why. Does it make you look tired or sallow? See what happens when you apply more blusher than usual. Does it clash with your natural skin tones? Try a slightly different shade of foundation makeup. Does it overpower you? Then use it in small doses—in a sweater or blouse, for example, not in a dress or coat.

Another trick for wearing a color that you love, but which you feel doesn't look well on you, is simply to keep that color away from your face. A magenta blouse, for example, may not be the greatest with your skin tones. But if you fill in the neckline with a scarf—one in a color that *is* flattering, magenta *can* be for you.

Another thing: at some point, after you have all the basics and are beginning to add more to your wardrobe, you probably should take pattern—prints, stripes, checks, plaids, etc.—into consideration. Specifically, decide for yourself whether you prefer pattern in your tops or your bottoms.

Some women tend to keep pattern on the bottom. Most of their sweaters, shirts, and blouses are in solid colors, while many of their pants and skirts are checks or plaids or prints. That way, while they undoubtedly have certain favorite combinations, they can still wear almost any top with any skirt or pair of pants. Other women prefer striped, printed, or plaid tops and solid-color skirts or pants, an approach that can be just as versatile as the first.

The point is this: if you don't make some kind of basic decision about whether you want pattern in your tops, or bottoms, you run the risk of ending up like the woman with an enormous collection of floral print blouses and a whole closetful of expensive tartan plaid skirts. Despite all the clothes she has from which to choose, she hardly looks really well dressed—for obvious reasons.

How to Shop Wisely and Well

For some women, going in and out of stores, looking at, trying on, and buying clothes is a wonderful way to spend the day. I know a few women who don't do much of anything *but* shop during the day. I'm not like that. Though I don't have a full-time nine-to-five job, I'm as busy as many women who do. And on those rare days when I'm not planning a fund-raising event for charity, or doing volunteer work, I'd much rather stay home and catch up on my reading, or do my bookkeeping, write thank-you notes, or take a tennis lesson than trudge around from store to store shopping for clothes.

The interesting thing, at least for me, is that so many of the chronic shoppers I know are the very same women who are constantly complaining that they have nothing to wear. It isn't exactly true, of course. They have closets full of clothes. But despite all their shopping, they just haven't built up a wardrobe.

The difference between them and me is that they shop in a scattered, disorganized way, while over the years I've built an extensive wardrobe. I really don't *need* to shop much anymore. As I mentioned earlier, I'm still wearing some of the things I bought twelve to fifteen years ago. But because they're so well made, because they suited me at the time and they still suit me, because there was nothing faddish about them to begin with, they're just as wearable now as they were when I bought them. (Especially the Norells I've collected over the years. They *never* go out of style. Recently I gave a hundred old Norells to the Costume Institute at the Metropolitan Museum of Art. They were having trouble finding Norells for the collection. Everybody just keeps on wearing the ones they have. Often, a friend will comment on a "new" skirt or dress I'm wearing and just can't believe it when I insist it's not new at all, but a 1965 Norell, or whatever.)

Scatter shopping—picking up a blouse here, an unrelated skirt there, and somewhere else a pair of pants that go with nothing in your closet—is very different from building a wardrobe.

Happening upon some marvelously attractive little shirt or a pair of unusually pretty shoes and then buying them on impulse—this can be one of life's small joys. Especially when the price is right. (I like a bargain as much as anyone.) Some of my very favorite things to wear are things I just "stumbled" upon when I least expected to, things I wasn't looking for and really didn't need until I saw them, loved them, and bought them.

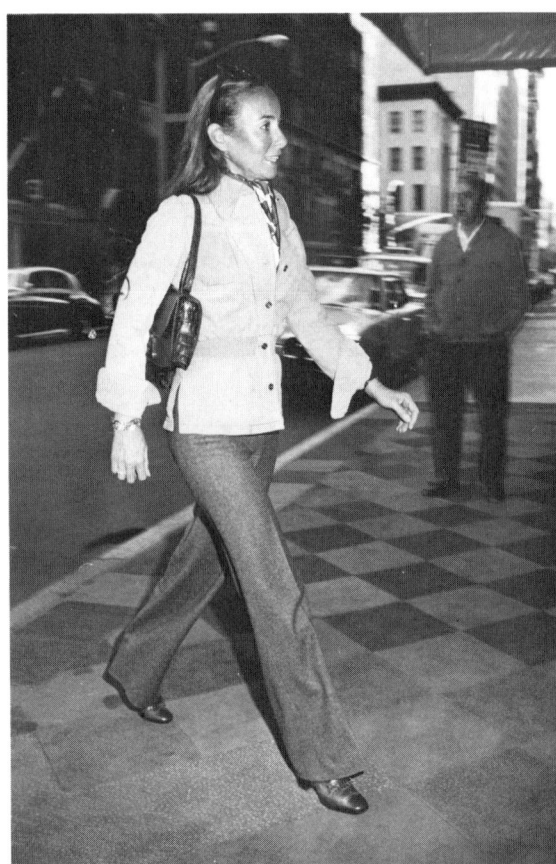

Clothes you love are never out of style. Everything that I'm wearing in the picture—the suede jacket, the gray flannel pants, the purse—is at least six years old. (PHOTO: WWD)

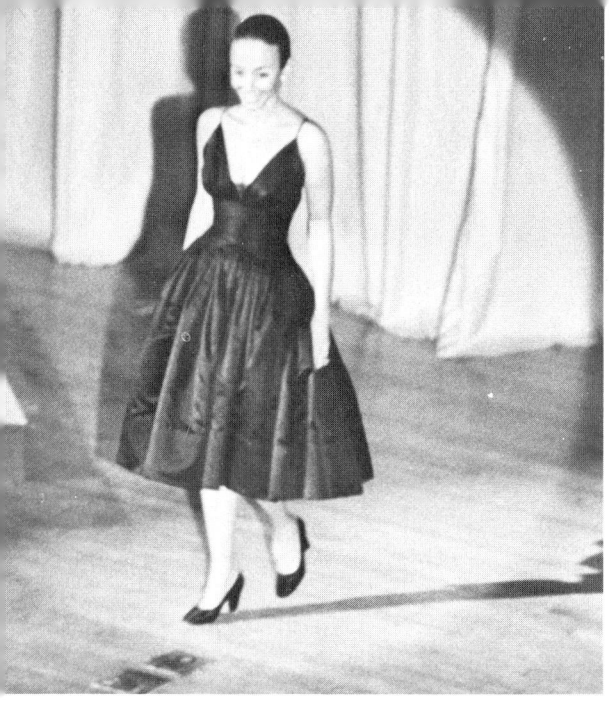 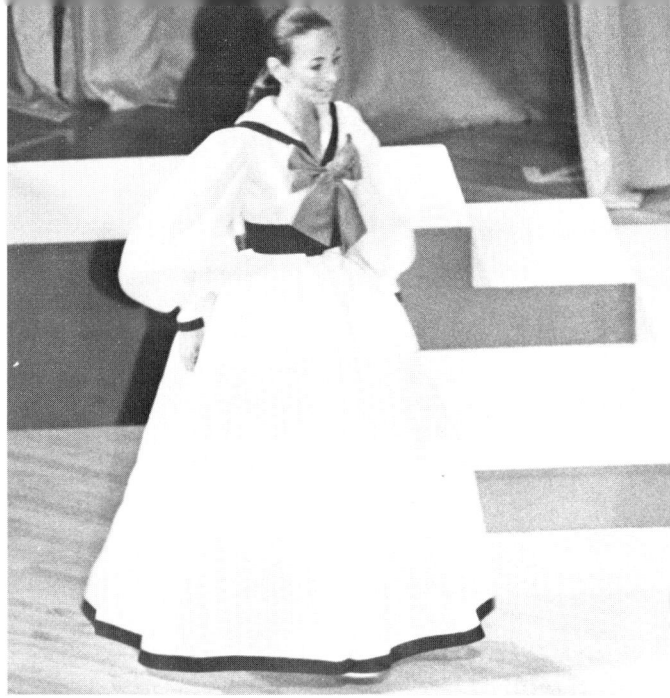

At the Norell retrospective show at New York's Metropolitan Museum: my first Norell (from way back when I was 17!); the famous Norell sailor dress; a collection of the sensational "drop dead" Norell beaded "sweater" dresses. (PHOTOS: KEVIN DUNCAN)

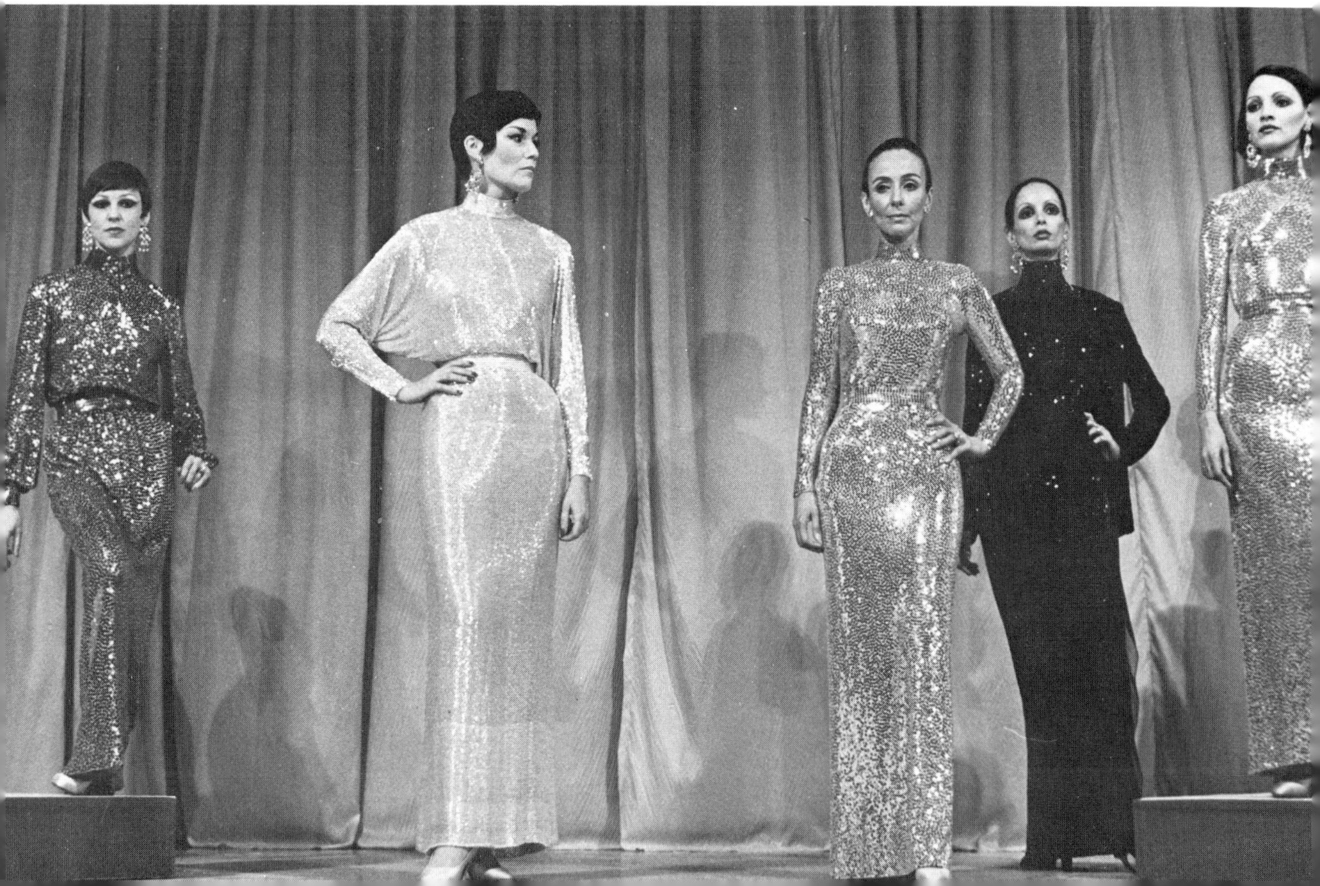

However, I'm aware that if I did all my shopping that way, buying on impulse without giving a thought to replacing or building on what I already have—without *planning,* in short—I'd be just like those others, always complaining about not having a thing to wear.

The way to be well dressed is to get your basics together, adding a major piece or two—a skirt or pants one season, perhaps a jacket or coat the next—as you need them and can afford them.

Over the years I've developed a way of adding to my own wardrobe—you might almost call it a "technique"—that might be helpful to you.

It's as simple as being aware of what's already in your wardrobe, as well as what's missing; knowing what you need (or want) and then buying it when you see it. In other words, no procrastinating.

If you see a really smashing pair of espadrilles, and you know you'll need (or want) espadrilles next summer, don't talk yourself out of them just because it's only November. Next summer will be here sooner than you think, and you may never find another pair of espadrilles that you like as well. The same goes for coats, suits, bathing suits, and anything else. When you see something, and it's right for you, and you know you'll be needing it someday—even if you won't actually be wearing it for months—snap it up if you possibly can.

I realize that from a money point of view, this may not always be possible. You might unexpectedly discover *the* dress for next summer on a blustery February day when you've left your checkbook or credit cards at home. Or it may be that at the moment your budget just can't stretch enough to accommodate the dress.

What do you do then? Well, I know what I'd do in such a situation. I'd write down the name of the manufacturer of the dress and where the company is located. (Ask a salesperson if you can't find the information on the label or hang tag.) That way, if the store was sold out of the dress by the time I was in a position to buy it, I could write to the manufacturer for the names of other stores that might still have it. So what if you're a New Yorker, and you have to order it from a store in Houston? Assuming the dress is exactly what you need or want, the extra effort will be worth it.

(You might also want to ask one of the salespeople to let you know when and if the dress is going to go on sale. You'd be surprised at how helpful the salespeople at some of the better stores can be.)

To illustrate my "technique" in action, let me tell you about a situation that arose a few weeks ago. Jimmy Galanos was in town, and on the spur of the moment I decided to run over to his suite at the Plaza. He was showing some wonderful street-length dresses for spring and summer. There was one in particular that I loved: full-skirted, with a wide belt, long sleeves, square neckline. Jimmy had done it in beige silk with tiny red stripes (like men's shirting fabric). At the time I went up there, I was aware that next fall I'd be needing a street-length dress for the ballet and restaurants. Since I was so pleased with the way the beige silk was made, I asked Jimmy if he could have another made for me in black crepe for next fall. He agreed.

I could have waited for fall to find the perfect dress. But as I've said, I'm not a shopper, and ordering from Jimmy on the spot saved me from having to look around later on. Also, how could I be sure I'd find another dress in a style that I'd like as well? So, know what you need and buy it when you see it.

I have another trick or two that can save you shopping time and even money. It has to do with ordering things in quantity, preferably when they're on sale. For eighteen years I've been wearing the same style bra, made by Hollywood Vassarette. Every couple of years I call Bloomingdale's and order more bras—usually ten white and two black at a time. I don't have to think about bras again for a long, long time.

I do the same thing with stockings, buying two dozen pairs every January from Bergdorf's. I always buy the sandalfoot kind (I don't know about you, but I find they don't run or snag any faster than the ones that have reinforcements at the heel and toe; their big advantage is that you can wear them with any shoe) in the darkest beige to make my legs look tan all year round. I'm also very lucky to know George Abbott, who makes all the pantyhose for J. C. Penney. (Incidentally, these are the best pantyhose I've ever worn. They're a good fit for my legs, neither too tight, nor big and baggy, and they're very, very sheer. He makes hose in all colors and in at least a half a dozen styles,

88 / *Lyn Revson's World of Style*

including the kind that come just up to the knee and are perfect for wearing with pants. And at about $1.29 a pair, the pantyhose are only a fraction of the price of Hanes or Dior's. I'm really not saying all of these nice things because he sends them to me for nothing. If I didn't think they were great, I wouldn't wear them.)

I even buy bathing suits in quantity. I get mine from Giorgio Sant'Angelo. I buy three or four at a time, not all the exact same style, but always the one-piece kind, which I think are the most flattering and sexiest of all. Most of his suits come with a skirt, so I'm not buying just a bathing suit but a whole beach outfit. (That's something

One-piece bathing suits, for me, are the sexiest of all. This one, by Giorgio Sant'Angelo has its own skirt (*right*) and becomes an instant outfit for luncheon by the pool, etc. (PHOTOS: LEE GUBER)

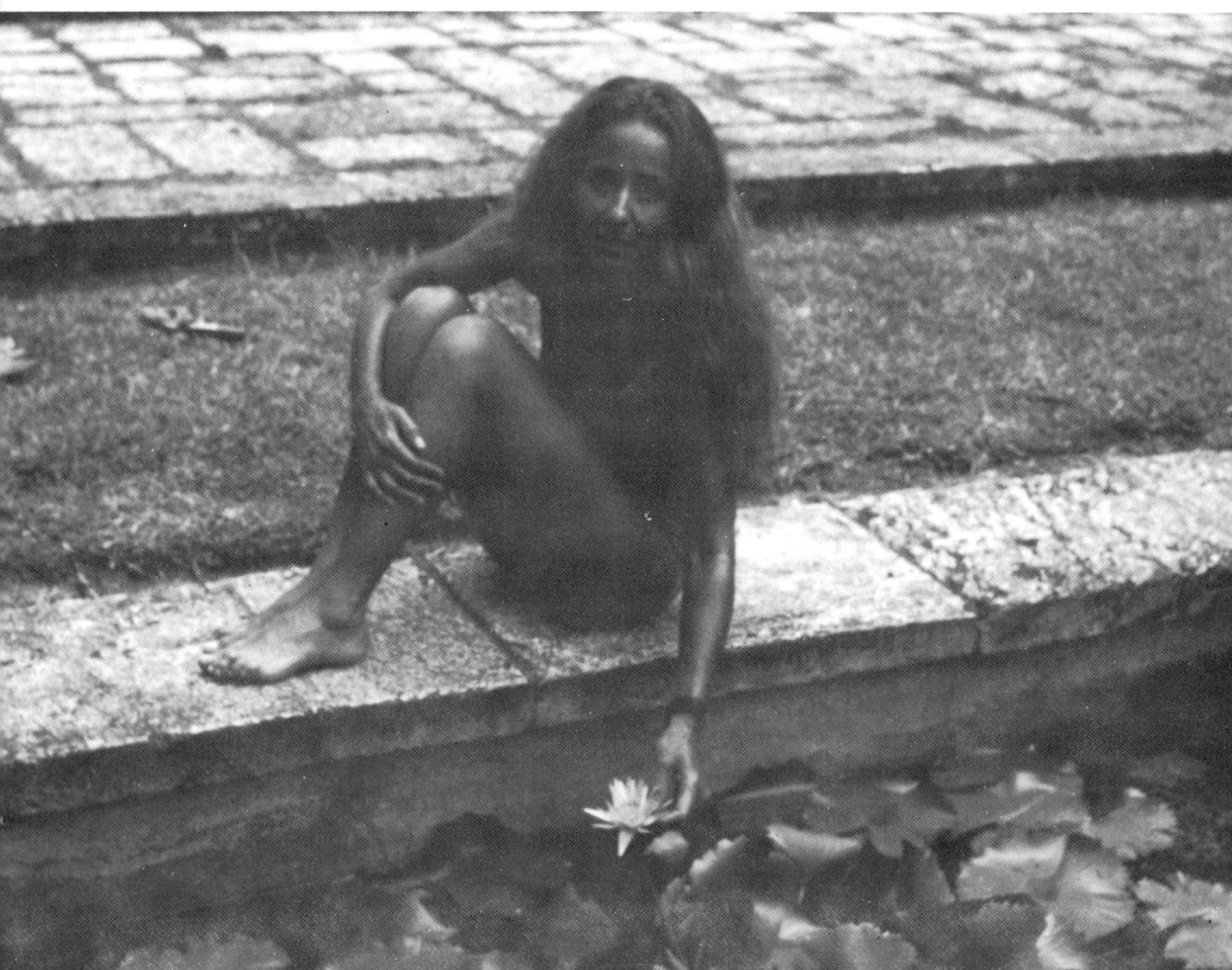

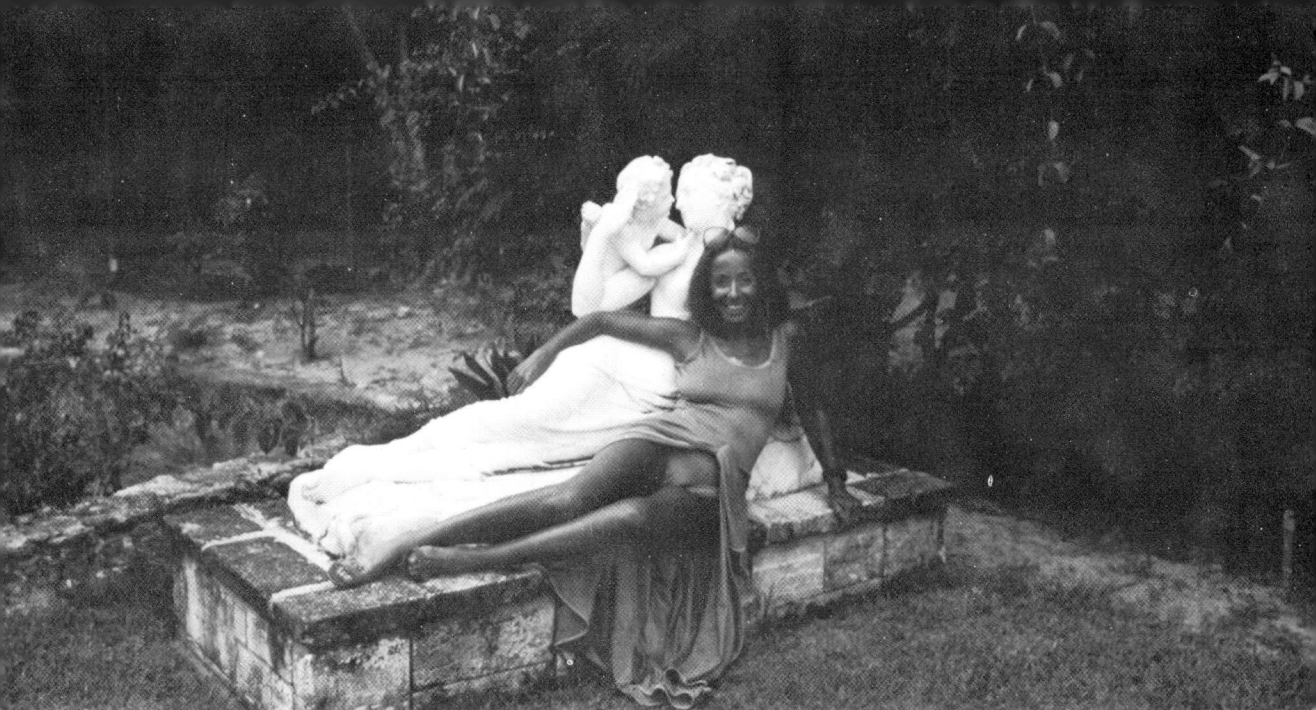

else you might want to keep in mind.) I also have three or four of his jumpsuits with plaid ribbon trim that are great to have in a wardrobe.

Finally, don't forget that many good stores have a personal shopping service that you can use at no extra charge. You can call the service, tell them what you're looking for, and they'll let you know whether they have it or not. You don't need to be specific about a manufacturer's name or style number. Just say you want a basic black dress with long sleeves and a high neckline (or whatever) and the personal shopper will tell you if the store has anything like it in stock. Using a store's personal shopping service may not save you money, but it could save hours of your time.

Judy Kroll, at Bloomingdale's, is the greatest. My friend Lee Guber, who produced *The King and I,* wanted to get Yul Brynner a black terry cloth robe as an opening-night present. (Yul *always* wears black—black shirts, black jackets, black pants.) Lee called everywhere. In all New York City, there was no such thing as a black terry cloth robe. Finally, he called Bloomingdale's and Judy Kroll had one made up within four hours!

What to Wear Where

I think it's always better to be a bit underdressed than overdressed. If you're going to err (I feel a little uncomfortable talking about "erring" here, because I truly believe that if it makes you happy to wear something, you're not making a mistake), you should err on the side of dressing down. In other words, if you're trying to decide between a rather elaborate cocktail dress and a silk shirt, skirt, and jeweled belt, you're probably better off wearing the latter.

The one exception is when you're dressing for a very large, very formal party or ball. That's when you really want to sparkle; otherwise, how are you going to stand out in the crowd? This is another piece of advice that came to me from the master, Norman Norell, and I'm convinced that he's absolutely right. I have several long, dark wool crepe dresses that are covered up and fairly subdued. I always enjoy wearing them. But when I'm going to a gala affair where there will be hundreds of people, I slip into something really sensational. One of my favorites comes from Norell. It's a close-fitting floor-length dress entirely covered with pink sequins. It's six years old, and it's still one of the greatest "grand entrance" dresses in town. (I have another, a gold one, that is eleven years old, and I still wear it.)

I know it's all very well for me to say "dress to the hilt" for the big gala occasions and "underdress" the rest of the time. But "underdressing" could mean practically anything—and these days it often does. Would you believe mechanic's coveralls at the opening night of last year's New York City Ballet season? Well, I wouldn't have, until I saw it with my own eyes.

Obviously, mechanic's coveralls at opening night at the ballet isn't quite what I mean by "underdressing." The woman who wore coveralls was underdressed, but she wasn't dressed appropriately.

The days when there were hard rules about what to wear where are gone, probably forever. That's basically a good thing. But it's still important to dress appropriately.

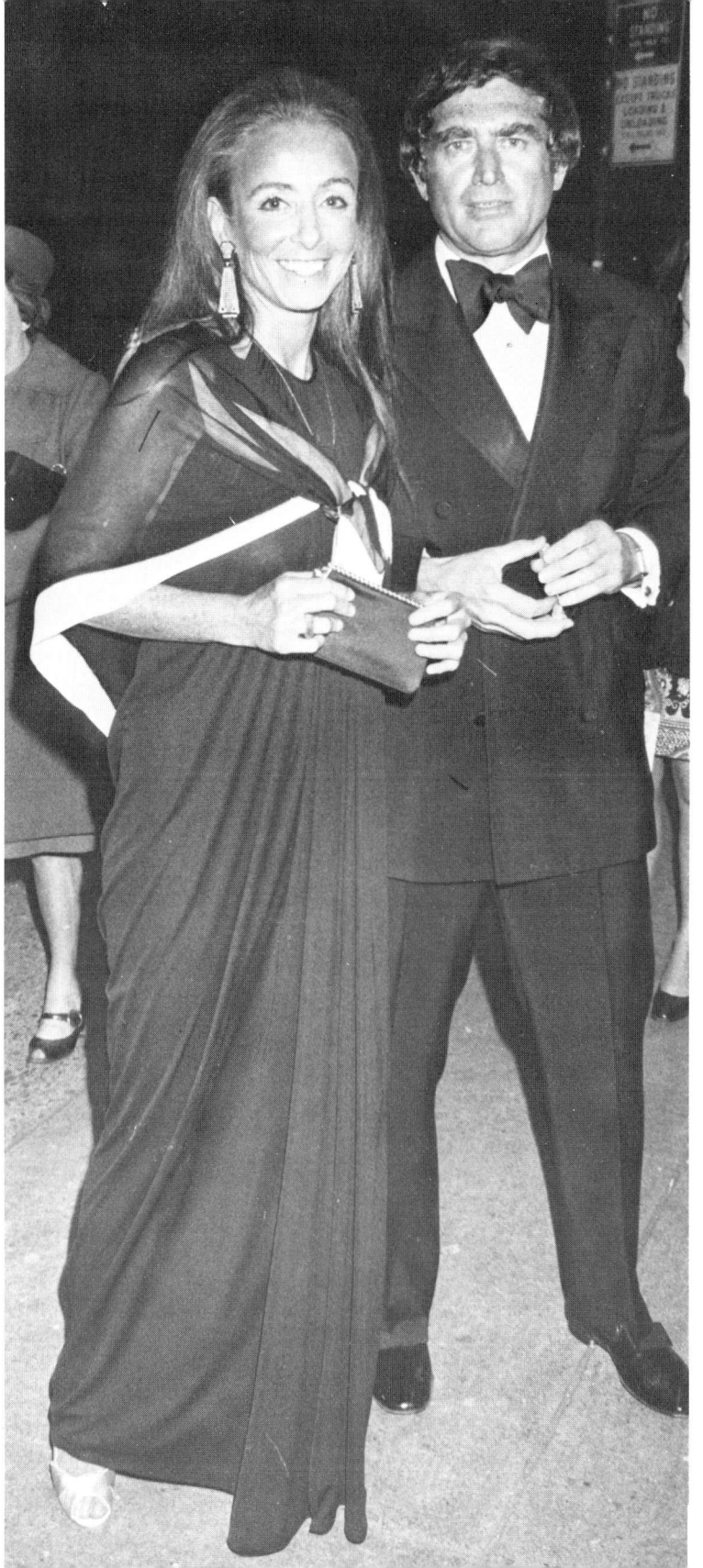

The black crepe dress (by Galanos) at a theater opening. My escort is Lee Guber.
(PHOTO: SAL TRAINA/WWD)

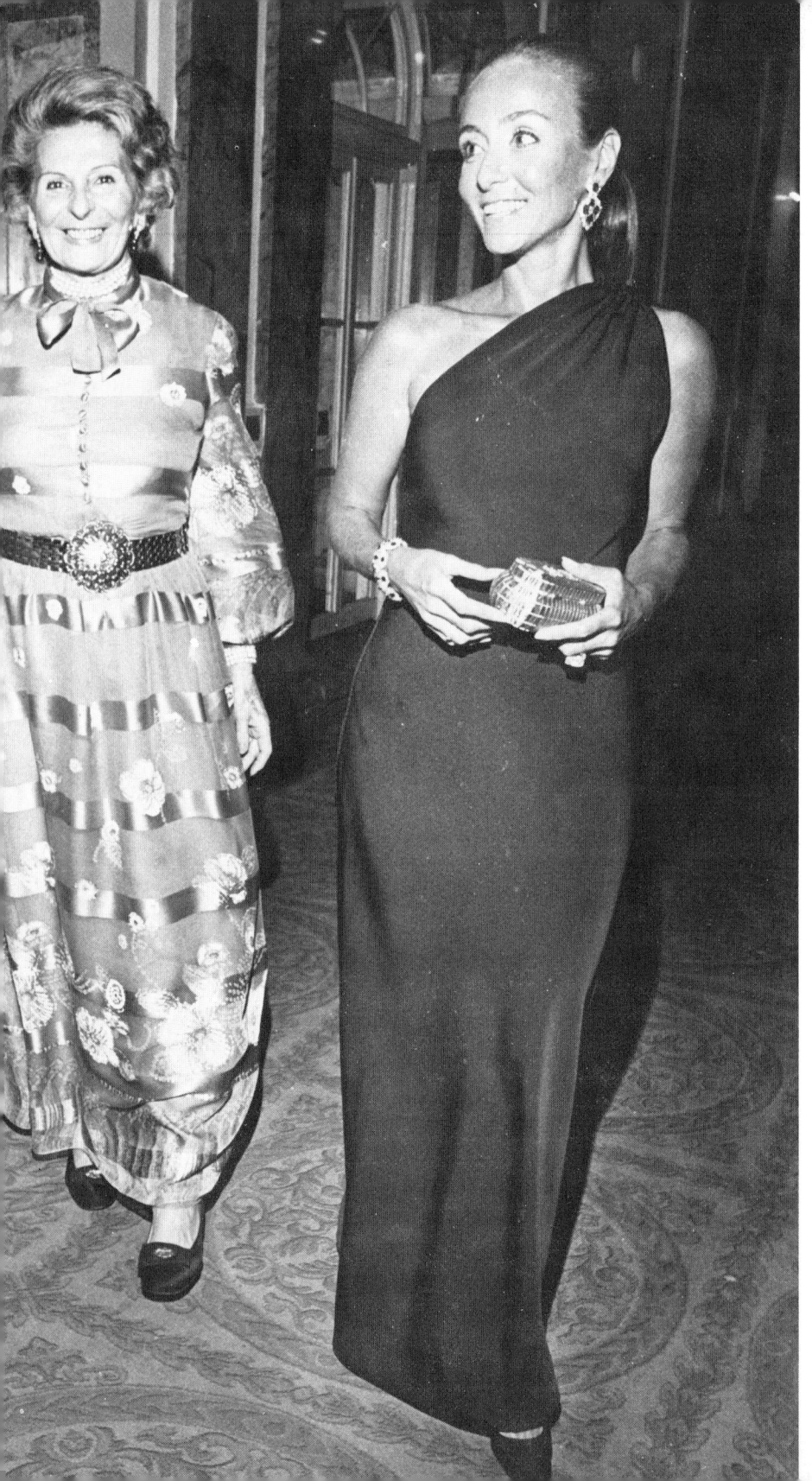

At a charity ball with Princess Marcella Borghese, I'm wearing a black silk-crepe Galanos dress. It's six years old, and such a favorite of mine that I have it in white too. In my hand I'm holding a gold minaudière, the "shrimp basket," designed by Jean Schlumberger of Tiffany.

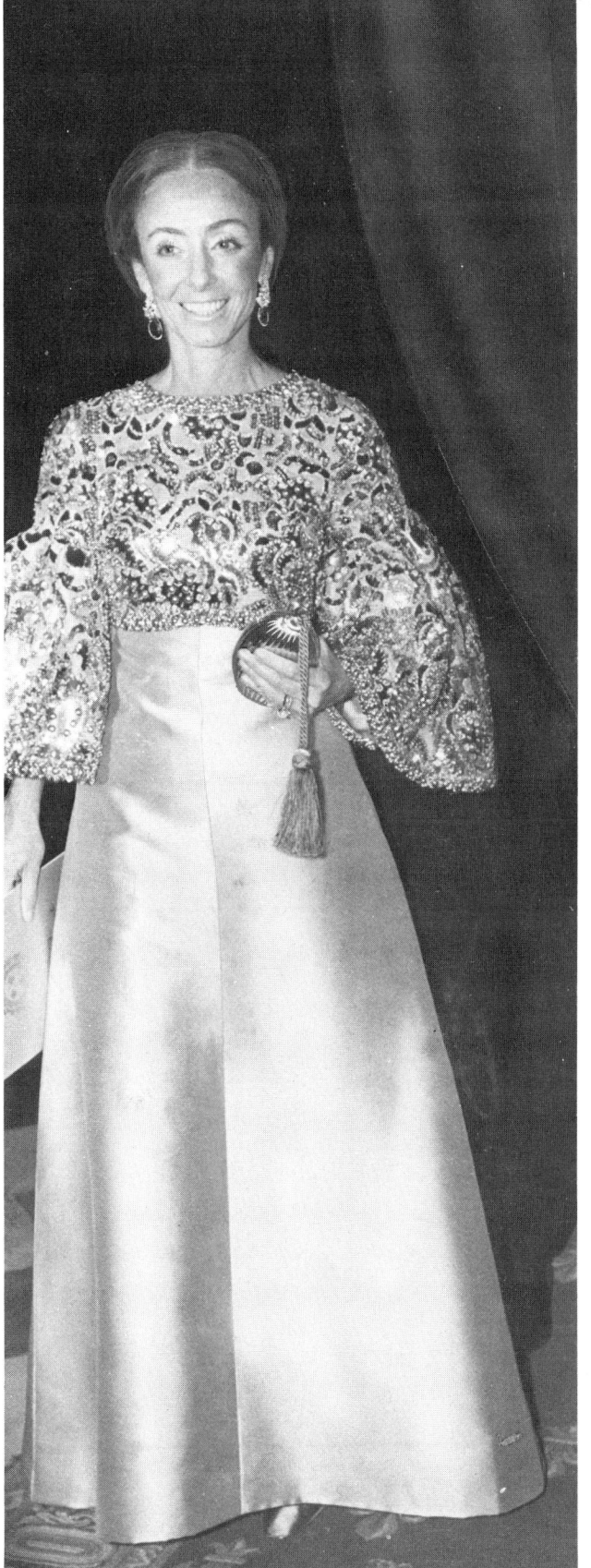

The larger the gathering and more festive the occasion, the more spectacular should be the dress. For the 1974 Versailles Ball I chose peach silk with heavily embroidered bodice and sleeves by Pierre Balmain. Alexandre gathered my hair into a chignon.

What makes one outfit appropriate while another is just plain wrong? It's mainly a matter of using your head. Common sense. Mechanic's coveralls are appropriate for gardening, painting the house, painting a picture, or tinkering with a car—but not for a ball or the ballet. A little black dress is appropriate for the theater, a restaurant, a gallery opening, but not for playing tennis or a day at the beach. It has to do with comfort and function.

It also has to do with your feelings about the people and the occasion for which you're dressing. One of the surest ways to get the message across that you don't give a damn about the people or the occasion is to dress inappropriately.

Take the woman who wears a bright pink denim sport skirt, cotton T-shirt, and beach scuffs to the funeral of her husband's boss. Unless her true feelings about the occasion run along the lines of "Whoopee, he's finally kicked off" (and she doesn't care who knows it), she's inappropriately dressed. Presumably, we go to funerals to indicate sadness or respect for the dead person and his or her family. Gay colors and lighthearted casual styles reflect a gay, lighthearted mood that is out of place at a funeral.

What *is* appropriate at a funeral? Well, unless you and the deceased had a close personal relationship, there's certainly no need to wear a black dress and veil. But it is preferable to wear clothes that reflect the gravity of the occasion. A neutral-colored cloth coat, or fur coat, over a skirt and blouse, or a wool dress of almost any color is fine. In warm weather, a simple dress—perhaps a T-shirt dress—again, in almost any color, is appropriate. I would avoid riotous prints or very bright pastels. (Another quirk of mine: recently, the pants suit has been turning up at funerals. Although there's nothing utterly "wrong" about wearing a nicely tailored pants suit on such an occasion, I couldn't bring myself to do it.)

It used to be that only a black dress and a hat would do at a funeral. Anything else was breaking the rules. But since most of those rules *are* a thing of the past, and with people turning up at funerals in golf shorts and other people getting married in blue jeans, it's no wonder so many women have such a hard time trying to figure out what to wear. Not just to funerals and weddings but to all the other big and little business and social functions we all have to dress for.

When I started to write this section, I realized that over the last few years I've been dealing with this problem by applying a few informal guidelines of my own—guidelines that simply *evolved.* They've helped me solve some of my own what-to-wear-where dilemmas. Perhaps they'll be helpful to you.

What to Wear to a Wedding: First, consider where and when it's going to be held. For a morning wedding in a church, synagogue, or at City Hall, you can't go wrong in a simple daytime dress or suit. Cotton or linen are good for summer, and any color or print is fine, except for white. (Maybe I'm old-fashioned, but I still believe that at a wedding, white is for the bride only.) A bare dress with a stole, or one with its own jacket, is a good choice because you can remove the cover-up for a slightly more dressed-up look at the reception afterward. The same goes for a winter wedding that takes place in the morning, except that you should be dressed more warmly—in wool, wool jersey, or heavyweight silk.

A good-looking, beautifully tailored pants suit that you can dress up with a silk blouse is perfectly okay at a morning wedding (though I prefer a dress or skirt, myself). But no denim, please, and nothing that looks like work clothes. I wouldn't wear flowing silk or chiffon pajamas either—nighttime looks are out of place at daytime functions.

For a wedding held outdoors in a garden or park or near a pool, I'd definitely wear a dress—probably one with a full, floaty skirt. My feeling is that most suits and pants suits are too tailored and "citified" for an outdoor wedding. If it were a "blue jean" wedding, I might wear crepe pants, silk shirt, and espadrilles.

Evening weddings are, as a rule, either white tie or black tie. Usually one or the other will be indicated on the invitation. Occasionally, an invitation will arrive saying "black tie optional."

"White tie," "black tie," and "black tie optional," of course, refer to what the men are expected to wear. We women are supposed to take our cue from them.

"White tie" translates to formal evening dress, with the men in tuxedoes or dinner jackets—and white-tie, of course—and the women in long gowns. A white-tie occasion is supposedly the most formal and "dressed up" of all. It's a time for elegant, rich fabrics, decolletage, furs and jewels if you have them. But I wouldn't worry too much if you don't. A simply covered-up gown worn with a strand of pearls, or flowers in your hair will do very nicely.

"Black tie," according to the dictionary, indicates "semiformal" evening attire. Nowadays, no matter what the dictionary says, there's very little difference between white tie and black tie. "Black tie" still means formal dress for the men—but not necessarily tails, and with a black bow tie instead of the white. And for women, a long gown is still best. From time to time I see evening pajamas worn at black tie weddings, but I generally avoid them. It's so much more fun to dance in a dress.

"Black tie optional" means semiformal or not, as you prefer. Men can choose from tuxedo or dinner jacket, or dark blue business suit; women can wear a long gown or long skirt and shirt; or a dressed-up street-length skirt and shirt, suit, or dress.

Incidentally, more and more invitations these days say "dress informal." This is not to be confused with "casual" dress and if you should receive one of these invitations, I wouldn't advise jeans and a T-shirt. A recent party at the home of Senator and Mrs. Jacob Javits was a perfect example of what "dress informal" means, at least in New York: all of the men wore business suits while the women were dressed to the hilt.

I think this new category arose mainly because there are far fewer balls than there used to be, but most women have formal clothes and they want to get dressed up occasionally. Most men, on the other hand, dislike getting into a tuxedo or dinner jacket and won't do it if they can possibly get away with wearing a business suit instead. (A pity, since so many of them look so well in formal clothes.) "Dress informal" keeps everybody happy.

I'd apply the above rules for weddings also to bar mitzvahs and most other evening occasions, including balls and dinner dances—in fact, to any nighttime event where the invitation specifies "white tie," "black tie," "black tie optional," or "dress informal." And, oh yes, don't forget what Norell had to say about dressing according to the size of the gathering: the larger the group, the more spectacular your dress, the better to stand out in the crowd.

COCKTAIL PARTIES: In New York and many other cities, the cocktail party has all but disappeared; more and more, people are entertaining at big and little dinner parties. (I'm not quite sure why except that many people feel that early evening is an inconvenient time of day for socializing and would rather get together later on for dinner; there's also the feeling that the dinner party lends itself better to interesting conversation than the overcrowded, noisy atmosphere of the typical cocktail party.) However, I know that the cocktail party lingers on in other parts of the country and dressing for one continues to throw some women into a quandary—especially women who have nine-to-five jobs and can't get home to change before the party.

I know what I'd do if that were my problem. In the morning, I'd put on a skirt and a silk blouse layered over a turtleneck. I'd top it with a velveteen jacket. Before I left for the office, I'd tuck some gold chains and a pair of high-heeled shoes into my bag. Then at five o'clock I'd "change" for the party. Off would come the turtleneck and my comfortable medium-heeled shoes. On would go the chains and the high-heeled shoes. Then I'd brush my hair, check my makeup, and go off and enjoy myself at the party.

The point is this: cocktail parties are usually short and come at an awkward hour. Dressing for one often *must* depend on where you've been before the party, and/or where you're going afterward. So, even though manufacturers continue to make "cocktail" dresses, you don't have to wear one to a cocktail party. With the exception of jeans or work clothes on the one hand, and a formal ball gown on the other, practically anything goes.

DINNER AND OTHER EVENINGS OUT AT SOMEONE'S HOUSE: These can be the most puzzling evenings of all to dress for. The hostess is sure to say that dress is "informal" or that you should wear "whatever you like." However, don't forget that "informal dress" may mean that all the women will turn up in long, formal gowns. Ask the hostess to be more specific if she says "informal." Does she really mean "casual?"

Here are a few more factors to keep in mind when you're trying to gauge the formality or informality of the evening.

First, parties and dinners given "in honor" of someone—these include birthday and anniversary parties, parties to welcome a new couple to the neighborhood or club, or to celebrate someone's promotion or other career accomplishment—all tend to be more dressed up than the party given for no particular reason. The same is true of the first party given in a new house or apartment. (A "housewarming," in other words.)

Large parties, especially large parties where many of the guests are unacquainted with one another, tend to be more formal than smaller ones.

A party in the city will almost always be more dressed up than a party given at someone's country or beach house.

So, at an anniversary party with seventy-five guests, I'd probably wear a long matte jersey dress, one from Galanos, because his are important without being fussy.

At a dinner party for twelve friends, in the city, I might choose a short chiffon dress or a simple wool evening dress.

At a get-together at someone's beach house, for eight people who know each other well, I'd wear a long T-shirt dress or white cotton pants and T-shirt. (My favorite T-shirt has a Pisces fish on it.)

At most parties I end up wearing either pants or a long dress. And by pants, I don't mean jeans. (I practically never wear them to someone else's house, though I live in jeans at my own.) I do mean well-tailored pants of wool, silk crepe, or for informal summer evenings, cotton duck.

An easy, elegant look that is a standby for me for an informal dinner at the home of friends is a silk shirt, wool pants (or silk or linen pants when the weather is warm), gold chains, and perhaps a shawl or a colorful sweater or jacket thrown over the shoulder. (You could substitute a long skirt for pants and the look would have the same kind of casual elegance.) When I want to be more dressed up, I wear a long dress, bare in the summer, covered up, with long sleeves, in the winter.

Pants, incidentally, are not always less dressed up than a long skirt or dress. Not when the pants are in an unusually rich or eye-catching fabric. I have two pairs of pants that are beaded all over—one in black and the other in silver. They were given to me by Norell eight years ago. When I wear either pair, I feel *very* dressed up indeed. (I wore the black ones to a housewarming at the new home of Pat Collins and Joe Raposo. It was a toss-up between black wool pants and the much more dressed-up beaded ones, but the beaded pants won out because, first, it was a large party, a housewarming, and quite an important occasion, and second, I can wear wool pants just about anywhere but I don't often feel beaded pants are appropriate. With the pants I wore a black turtleneck sweater.)

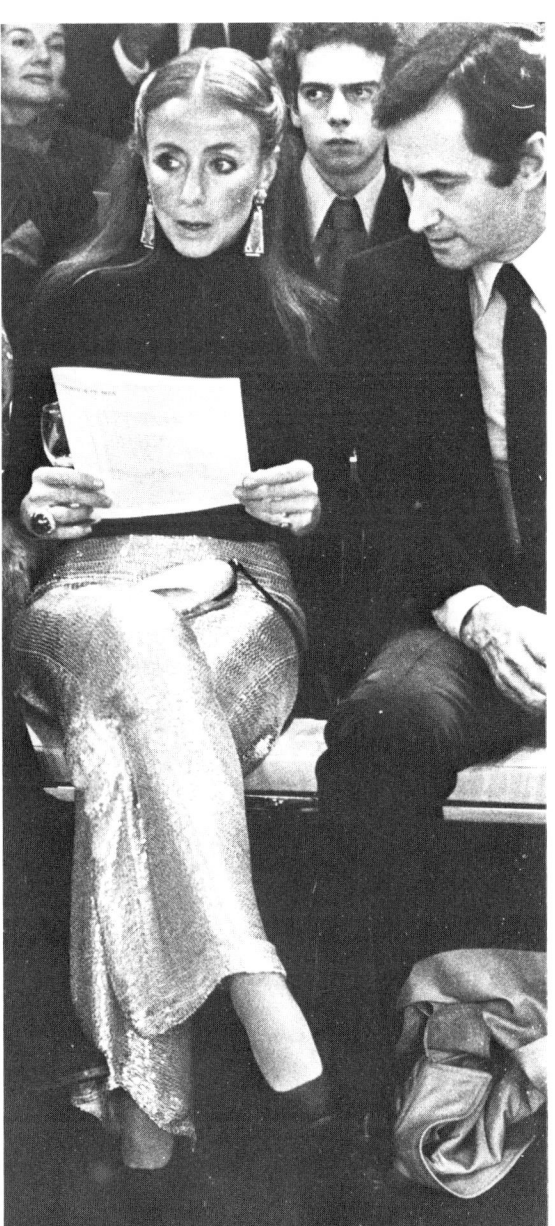

Norell's bugle-beaded pants, black cashmere turtleneck sweater, and black satin shoes (one has a red heel, the other a green heel) by David Evins. Alexandre did my hair earlier in the day. Here, I'm at an evening fashion show in Paris. (PHOTO: WWD)

In Acapulco one summer, at a party for eighteen on a yacht, I wore white wool pants, white silk shirt, a gold chain with a diamond lion pendant, and espadrilles with rubber soles (for a more secure footing in case the boat started to sway. I'm a big one for falling down, and if it weren't for my brilliant orthopedic surgeon and very good friend Dr. James Nicholas, I'd probably spend half my time in a wheelchair).

The white wool pants came from Hermès; the silk shirt was custom-made (I had it copied from a man's tuxedo shirt, pleated front and all), and David Evins made the brown alligator espadrilles especially for me. Jacqueline Onassis was there in a black evening gown and delicate high-heeled shoes. She looked lovely, but the shoes could have been a problem. At another yacht party, designer Mollie Parnis fell down a flight of iron stairs because she was wearing high-heeled shoes. (What a wonderful tough lady; she picked herself up and there wasn't a black-and-blue mark on her!)

Two looks I generally avoid when I go to a party or dinner at the home of friends are the daytime dress or suit and the flowing caftan. To me, most street-length dresses and suits, even the very same ones that are just the thing for a restaurant or the theater or other little evenings out on the town, feel out of place in the friendliness and intimacy of someone's home.

As for evening pajamas and caftans, like hostess gowns they've always seemed to me to be "at-home" clothes, better suited to the woman who's giving the party than the one who is there as a guest. (Again, my reluctance to wear "at-home" clothes to a party at someone's house has nothing to do with any "rule" of dressing; it's simply a reflection of the way I feel about the matter. Many well-dressed women *do* wear caftans, evening pajamas, and other clothes with an "at-home" feeling to parties and dinners given by their friends.)

Now, what do you wear to your own dinner or party? To begin with, don't forget that as hostess you're not only the one who decides the guest list and the menu, you're also the one who determines the degree of formality and sets the whole mood of the evening. What you wear should reflect what you want the party to be.

If you want a very informal get-together of close friends, where good food and good talk are the order of the evening, then by all means tell your guests exactly what you have in mind—don't say "informal" if you mean "casual"—and wear a T-shirt and blue jeans, if that's what you feel like wearing. (I do it all the time.)

Or perhaps you're planning a more formal evening—say, a sit-down dinner for twenty to celebrate the wedding anniversary of a pair of dear friends. You'll want to look more "dressed" than you would at a very casual gathering of six or eight. Perhaps a long matte jersey dress would be a good choice.

Finally, one very important thing to keep in mind when you're planning what to wear as hostess. If you don't have help and will be doing much of the cooking and serving yourself, make sure to choose clothes that are not only attractive and appropriate but also allow you freedom of movement and won't get in the way of what you're doing. Watch out for blouses and caftans with sleeves so wide they get mixed in with the salad when you toss it. Avoid anything so tight that the seams are strained whenever you stretch or bend to peek into the oven. And if your hair is long, tie it back or wear it in a chignon.

A Few Fashions to Avoid

Though I've always tried to be open-minded and learn from people who really know what they're talking about, I also dislike the idea of anyone—expert or not—setting down a detailed list of fashion rules and expecting me or anyone else to follow them. After all, you and I are the ones who will be wearing the clothes we buy and if *we're* pleased with the way we look, what else really matters?

That's why all the suggestions I've made so far—with the exception of the section on building a basic wardrobe—have been offered with the hope that they'll give you a better idea of *how* to choose for yourself, not *what* to choose.

However, I do have a few rather strong opinions about some of the current fashion looks and I can't resist writing them down here, for whatever they may be worth.

I'll start with the designer-initial fashions—those belts, scarves, pieces of costume jewelry, handbags, and fabrics emblazoned with the initials (sometimes even the signature!) of the man or woman who designed them. I don't like these fashions at all.

For one thing, I'm not the least bit interested in wearing anyone's initials but my own. Certainly, I'm not willing to turn myself into a walking advertisement for someone's product, no matter how great the designer or the product. An advertisement is exactly what you become when you wear a designer's initials. (And to think that most businesses have to pay dearly for their advertising!)

What of the woman who *does* wear designer-initial scarves, belts, and so on? My first impression of her is always that she must be insecure about her own sense of style and that she wears these fashions to bolster her image as a person of taste. (It's the same kind of mentality that snips the original label from a new coat or dress and replaces it with a designer label—a practice that's more common than you might think.) Of course, it's possible that wearing designer-initial fashions may have nothing to do with insecurity. I'll also concede that a woman might buy the same item minus the initials, just because she likes it. But the vibes I get from these fashions and the women who wear them tell me otherwise.

Then there's the matter of matching. Every once in a while I see a woman who's obviously made an attempt to match her belt to her bag to her shoes, or her earrings to her necklace to her bracelets, or to pick up one of the colors in the print of her blouse and match to it her scarf, jewelry, skirt and/or tights. This kind of matching isn't necessary.

Not only that, too much matching calls attention to itself and looks contrived. It becomes a gimmick, and gimmicks are to be avoided.

I don't mean that if you have brown alligator shoes and a brown alligator handbag you shouldn't wear them together. Matching shoes with a bag is fine (though I personally would choose black or brown calf shoes with my alligator bag). But adding a brown alligator belt and an alligator watchband is going several steps too far.

The mark of true fashion savvy isn't matching. That's something I learned many years ago from my friend Marilyn Evins. It's coordinating. What's the difference? Well, in matching the idea is to put together identical colors or prints or textures so that various items of clothing and accessories seem to have been made of the same materials. In coordinating, the emphasis is on maintaining a certain style or mood or scale in a pleasing range of colors and textures.

If you still don't get what I mean, pick up almost any issue of *Vogue* and look through the color photographs. Notice how little (if any) matching there is. Instead, the colors, textures, mood, and scale of the clothes and accessories are complementary, and add up to a harmonious whole.

Another fashion no-no (for me at least) are clothes made of plasticky-looking man-made or synthetic fabrics. Some of the synthetics are attractive, of course. Ultrasuede, to name just one. But the disadvantages of many synthetics outweigh their advantages.

For one thing, synthetic fabrics tend to be nonabsorbent, which makes them feel rather clammy to the touch and uncomfortably hot to wear when the weather is warm.

That's not all. Many synthetic fabrics are processed to look like fabrics made of natural fibers such as wool, cotton, silk, linen. The trouble is, in many cases, the resemblance is a very poor one.

Of course, one of the big advantages of some of the synthetic fabrics is that they stay wrinkle-free and need little or no ironing after they've been washed. This makes them useful for children's play clothes, for sheets and pillowcases, tablecloths, napkins, and other items that get heavy use and need frequent laundering.

Another advantage is that many things made of synthetic fabrics— though not all—are less expensive than the same article made with natural-fiber fabrics.

But all in all, I feel about clothes made of synthetic fabrics the way I do about fake fur coats. A few, the ones that are *very* well made of high-quality synthetic materials, are attractive. As for the rest, I'll continue to avoid them. Why have something that's supposed to look and feel like wool or cotton (or silk or linen) when you can have the real thing instead?

Nonfunctional clothes are another category I generally avoid. Anything with buttons, snaps, or zippers that are so tricky (or so numerous) that I have a hard time getting in and out of it has no place in my closet. Tennis dresses in bright colors are another example: white is traditional because it's easy to see and reflects the sun. No other color works as well, yet nowadays it's a rainbow-colored fashion show on the tennis courts.

Boots in summer, especially in the city, are another example. I wear boots in the winter for warmth and to protect the backs of my legs from getting chapped and reddened by the cold. But indoors, even in the winter, boots are unnecessary—nonfunctional. And in the summer, it's downright masochistic to wear them.

Other items that fall into this category are ski clothes you can't ski in (because they're not waterproof, or they're too tight), raincoats that don't keep you dry, and well, need I go on? The stores are crowded with clothes that don't do the job they're supposed to do. Some of them may be attractive, but they're still bad fashion.

A Final Word about Money and Clothes

Way back at the beginning of this section I mentioned that you don't need to have a lot of money to be well dressed in a unique personal style.

Believe it or not, money can actually be a hindrance. If you have unlimited money to spend, you can afford to buy anything that strikes your eye without thinking twice about whether it's a good choice for you. There are no restraints.

With less money, you're forced to buy more carefully. Every purchase *has* to be a good one. If you learn how to make every dollar count, you may end up being far better dressed than the woman who has many times more money to spend on clothes than you do. I won't name names, but some of the women I know who spend fortunes—literally!—on clothes, don't dress as well as some of the working women I see on the streets every day.

Quality does count, of course. I've already explained why it's important to get the best-quality workmanship at the price you can afford to pay, and why a small, well-chosen basic wardrobe is better than closets crammed with clothes that don't work together.

The truth is, once you've established a fashion identity, it won't matter too much anymore what you pay for your clothes. A perfect example: I ran into someone on the street the other day, a friend of a friend. She went into ecstasies over my jeans. "They're sensational. Where did you get them? They have to be Norell."

Norell? Those jeans cost me $7.95 six years ago at Jax. I bought several pairs, and my son Steven bleached them out in the bathtub for me. I explained all this, but the woman refused to believe me. She knows I can afford to pay whatever I like for jeans and she was convinced that the ones I was wearing—nicely fitting and well made, to be sure—were something that they weren't. Not in the mood to argue about it, I just shrugged and changed the subject.

4

Friends and Other People

Style isn't just achieving a special, personal look in your clothes, your hair, and your makeup. Style is also knowing how to handle yourself in situations—especially situations involving other people.

It is, among other things, knowing how to cultivate friendships and business relationships without being pushy or manipulative. How to express warmth and interest in the people you already know, as well as the people you'd like to know better. How to make the most of your social time. How to accept invitations and how to know which ones to turn down. How to know when to send a gift, and how to choose just the *right* gift for the person and the occasion. Just as important, it's knowing how to do all of these things in ways that feel right and comfortable and that express your very *personal* style.

There's nothing mysterious or difficult about any of it. Learning to do these things, and doing them well, is, like almost everything else in life, a matter of using your head, practice, and confidence. You already know how to use your head. And the confidence comes with practice.

How to Cultivate People for Fun and Profit

A lot of people feel uncomfortable about the word "cultivate" when it's applied to human beings. They needn't. "Cultivating" is simply taking steps to form a relationship with a person you'd like to get to know, or get to know better. Every time you make an approach to someone you're interested in, either socially or for business reasons, you're attempting to cultivate that person. Everyone does it.

But some people don't know how to do it well. They try too hard. A perfect example is a woman I know who called to invite me to a party. When I told her I was sorry, I couldn't make it, I was going to the theater that night, she sounded very disappointed. We talked for a minute or two more, said good-bye, and I thought that was the last of it. But no, she called twice more, asking if I couldn't possibly change my plans and come to her party. On the third call, she said, "But you *must* come, I've told the others you'd be there."

You could say this woman was trying to "cultivate" me, but she'd gone about it in exactly the wrong way. It wasn't that I resented being invited to her party. Though I can't always accept an invitation, I'm almost always flattered to be asked. What annoyed me was her unwillingness to take no for an answer, her pushiness, her attempt to manipulate me.

Pushiness is part of a negative personal style. So is manipulation. I wouldn't want to recommend them to anyone. Being pushy or manipulative won't get you anywhere or win you anything except a reputation for being obnoxious.

Simpering and fawning and yessing people left and right usually don't work either. It's true, some people—even some "important" people—seem to need a "yes-person" and always have one on hand.

The yes-person builds them up and makes them feel more important. In return for always being flattering and agreeable, the yes-person has the privilege of being included in all the "important" person's social plans.

From the outside, the relationship might look like a close one. Even the yes-person might assume that it's a friendship. But if the yes-person stops yessing and begins to show signs of having a mind of her own, she gets dumped. I've seen it happen many times. The woman who chooses fawning and flattery as a way to get where she wants to be usually ends up playing the fool.

There's another, better way to cultivate people that often does work. It's part of a positive personal style that anyone can adopt. All it requires is the ability to express warmth and interest without overdoing it. That plus enough intelligence to keep your foot out of your mouth. If you can master these simple skills, you can cultivate just about anyone who's willing to be cultivated.

Expressing warmth and interest can be as simple as making eye-to-eye contact the first time you meet a person. It's listening when he or she talks. It isn't *always* agreeing with that person just for the sake of being agreeable. (You don't want to set yourself up for becoming a yes-person, do you?) At the same time, there's no reason to ridicule or belittle the other person's viewpoint because it doesn't jibe with your own.

You can express warmth and interest by inviting someone to lunch or dinner or a party at your house. (When I suggested this to someone, she threw up her hands. "But I hardly *know* them," she protested. "Well, what better way to *get* to know them?" was my answer.)

Remembering people at Christmas or on their birthdays or sending a little token gift "just because" (more about gifts later on) expresses warmth and interest. So does remembering their *children.* (I'm more inclined to like anyone who seems to be truly interested in my children. I suppose all mothers are that way.)

It goes without saying, but I'll say it anyway: it's foolish to disparage behind their backs the very same people you're attempting to cultivate when you're face-to-face. Word gets around. That's part of what I meant about having enough intelligence to keep your foot out

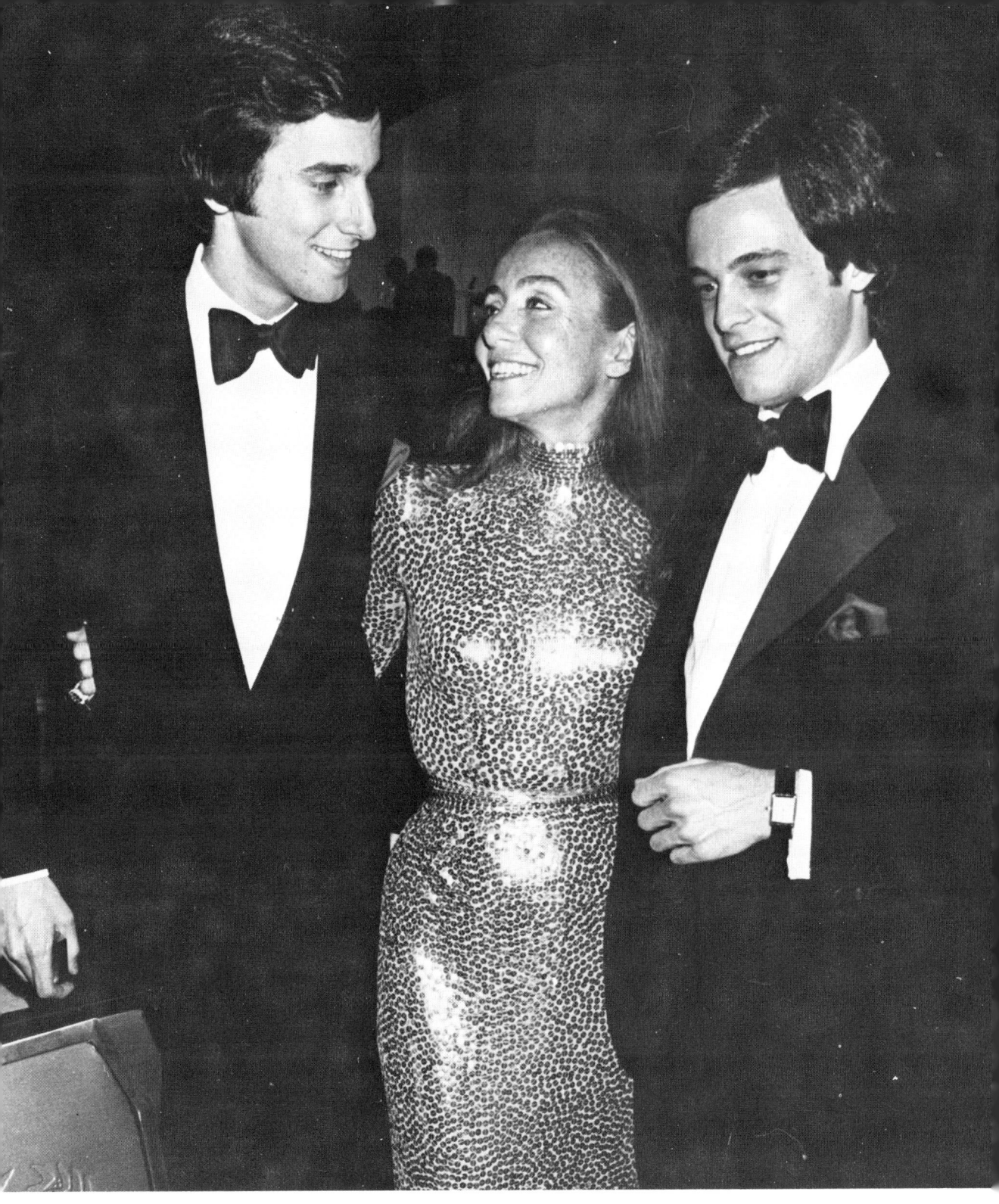

With my sons Jeffrey (left) and Steven, at a dinner in honor of Governor Hugh Carey of New York.

of your mouth. The other part has to do with simply having your wits about you—*thinking* before you speak.

Here's a woman who didn't think before she spoke:

A few years ago a friend asked me to be present while he talked with a man he was considering for a top position with a multimillion-dollar corporation. My friend was interested in getting to know the man's wife as well. (If the man was hired, his wife would be doing a certain amount of entertaining; on those occasions, she would act as a kind of unofficial representative of the company, so it was important that she be a person of at least *some* charm and style.)

The four of us were to meet at a restaurant. The other couple (I'll call them Mr. and Mrs. A) arrived a few minutes after my friend and I had been seated.

Mr. A, looking alert and confident, practically bounded over to our table. Mrs. A, carefully dressed but with a rather grim expression on her face, hung back slightly. She looked as though she wished she were someplace else—anyplace but in that restaurant under those circumstances. I put her very apparent uneasiness down to a simple case of the jitters. What woman wouldn't be somewhat nervous in a situation where a six-figure annual income for her husband might be hanging in the balance?

My friend, Mr. A, and I made small talk for a while. Mrs. A's contribution was mostly stony silence. As the conversation eventually swung around to the corporation and the job for which her husband was being considered, Mrs. A fiddled with the silverware and stared off into space. But when my friend mentioned something about the long hours everyone put in at the company, Mrs. A opened her mouth and made the definitive statement of the evening: "But we have dinner at six every night, and we've been doing it for fifteen years."

Stunned, Mr. A looked at his wife as though she'd dumped her soup in his lap. Nobody spoke for a moment. (Nobody knew what to say.) Then the talk went on to other things. Mr. A didn't get the job.

I honestly don't know whether he would have been offered the position if his wife had behaved otherwise. I do know that he would have had a better chance if his wife had made an attempt to present herself in the best, most favorable light she could manage instead of just sitting back like a wooden Indian—and then blurting out that absurd comment about dinner at six every night. (She couldn't have come up with a more damaging statement—not even if she'd racked her brains for hours beforehand.)

I've thought a lot about that incident—which I assure you is a true one. I don't understand Mrs. A's behavior. I have to conclude that she's stupid. One thing is certain: she doesn't know the first thing about cultivating people.

Invitations: When to Say Yes, When to Say No, and How to Say Either

How much easier our lives would be if deciding whether to accept certain invitations were the most difficult decisions we ever had to make. In the overall scheme of things, these decisions are minor in the extreme.

Yet they must be made, and usually they have to be made quickly. When an invitation arrives in the mail, you have a day or two to mull it over. When someone phones to invite you to a dinner or party you usually have to think fast.

In either case, of course, if your engagement book tells you that you've already committed yourself to someone else's party or dinner for that evening, there's no decision to be made. You simply pick up the phone (or tell the person waiting on the other end of the line) and say—regretfully, if you like—that you've made other plans.

There are very, very few utterly unforgivable social sins, but almost everyone I know agrees that accepting an invitation and then canceling out if something more fun or more "important" presents itself is one of them. Not that some people don't continue to do just that. Offhand, I can think of two or three couples who have more than once switched their evening plans when something more interesting came along—more interesting in their case apparently meaning more in line with their blueprint for social advancement. (How do I know? The world is always a much smaller place than we think it is. Word gets around.) These couples are rapidly gaining the reputation of being "climbers," and I doubt that it will be long before they no longer have the luxury of picking and choosing from among great numbers of invitations.

Rule number one, then, is this: refuse all invitations for evenings when you're already committed.

As for the other times, when the evening is open, there are no rules. But you needn't feel you *must* be available to anyone who calls or sends an invitation your way. That would be living under constant tyranny. Nor, in my opinion, is it wise to have a blanket policy of never going out in the evening if you can possibly avoid it. (Though I know some people who have such a policy and they tell me they like it better that way.) Perhaps the best way to decide whether or not to accept an invitation is to ask yourself, "What's in it for me?" And "What's in it for me?" turns out to be a two-part question: Will it be fun? Will it be useful?

Yes, I know, stated so boldly it does sound like a cold-blooded way to approach a social decision. Parties and dinners are supposed to be fun. At least it's always assumed that we go to them to enjoy ourselves and have a good time. But only the *very* naive don't also have an alternate view of social events: that they can be opportunities for making important business and social connections. (The difference between merely being aware of this and being a "climber" has to do with whether you allow the desire to make connections take precedence over basic consideration and tact.)

In any event, when you ask yourself "What's in it for me?" the decision is easier to make. If you think you'll have fun, say yes. If you doubt you'll really enjoy yourself but feel it will be to your social or business advantage to go, say yes. (And before you leave for the party, try to get in a more positive, "up" frame of mind. I believe that we're all at least partially responsible for making our own fun. I know myself that when I go someplace with the expectation of enjoying myself, very often I do.)

As for those obligatory events where your presence is absolutely required—the dinner in honor of a close friend, the surprise birthday party for your sister, almost any party given by your boss or your husband's boss—well, then you have no choice. Say yes. (And again, make up your mind to have a good time.)

Let's suppose you've accepted an invitation but something unforeseen happens, something that prevents you from going. You owe it to your hostess to let her know, as soon as possible, that you can't be there. Some people would disagree with me, but I also think you owe her a simple explanation: that one of your children is quite ill and needs you, that either you or your husband has a fever or the flu, that your work obligations have collided with your social commitments, etc. Nothing elaborate. Just a statement of facts.

What if you have a choice and you decide there's absolutely nothing in it for you to attend a particular social event? It shouldn't be a problem. Just say you're busy that evening and leave it at that.

You don't need to say *how* you're going to be busy. In fact, it's always best to keep things vague. Even though you may have an impulse to do so, it's not a good idea to quickly make up an engagement that doesn't exist. (It's too easy to get caught.) And long, involved explanations of how you think your mother-in-law may be in town that weekend, and if she is, you're going to have to go with her to the theater, or of how you've been feeling under the weather lately and you just don't know how you're going to be feeling in two weeks so to be on the safe side you'd better not plan on going—well, such explanations are not only unnecessary, they're very easy to see through. They also make it impossible for you to accept another invitation.

A simple refusal is always best.

How to Go Out "As Well as You Can"

My feeling has always been, about everything, if you're going to do it at all, get the most out of it and do it as well as you can. If I'm going out to a party or other social event, my nature is not just to sit there waiting to be entertained, but to throw myself into it, to make it an enjoyable evening for myself and for others, to go to the party "as well as I can." I feel that in accepting an invitation, I'm also accepting a kind of responsibility to do just that.

For me, going out "as well as I can" means meeting people at least halfway. It means looking alive. It means having something to say. It also means having some awareness of what not to say. It means enjoying myself as much as possible but not worrying about it if, despite my efforts, the evening is a dud.

I never gave much conscious thought to any of these things until it came time to write this book. Then I thought about them a lot. I realized that over the years, without ever being aware of it, I've been practicing certain "techniques." Perhaps some of them will be useful to you.

SMILING: Did you ever stop to realize that just smiling at people is a way of meeting them halfway? A smile says, "I'm glad to be here and I'm glad you're here, too." (A slightly different kind of smile says, "I'm glad to be here with *you.*") It also says, "I'm open to what's happening in this room [or at this table]. I'm interested. I'm alive."

A glum, bored, or disdainful expression says, "I'd rather be somewhere else. I'm wasting my time here. I wish to hell this whole thing were over with."

I don't know about you, but when I look around a room and see faces that register gloom, boredom, or disdain, I'm not intrigued. I don't want to know what's eating them. I certainly don't want to try to lift them out of their down mood. I wonder why they bothered to come at all. And I tend to gravitate away from them. (Faces like that are always a reminder to me to keep on smiling!)

The sad thing is, many people, especially shy, insecure people, purposely adopt a superior, above-it-all expression when they doubt their ability to get along well and have fun in a particular social situation. I'm not sure why, but I think it has something to do with trying to hide their shyness and insecurity. They'd rather give the impression that they're bored and above it all than risk smiling and looking too eager, "hungry" for attention and approval.

What they don't stop to consider is that the bored, above-it-all expression gets them nowhere. It doesn't make them look more interesting, more "with it"; it only makes them less appealing. The person who wants to camouflage shyness is much better off "hiding" it behind a smile.

EYE CONTACT: Like smiling, making eye contact is another important social device. Looking people directly in the eye lets them know you're interested in them—which in turn sparks their interest in you.

Many people, particularly shy, insecure people, find it very difficult to look others in the eye. So they focus on their drinks, or on the

With Eugenia Sheppard, fashion columnist, at a charity luncheon. (PHOTO: AL LEVINE)

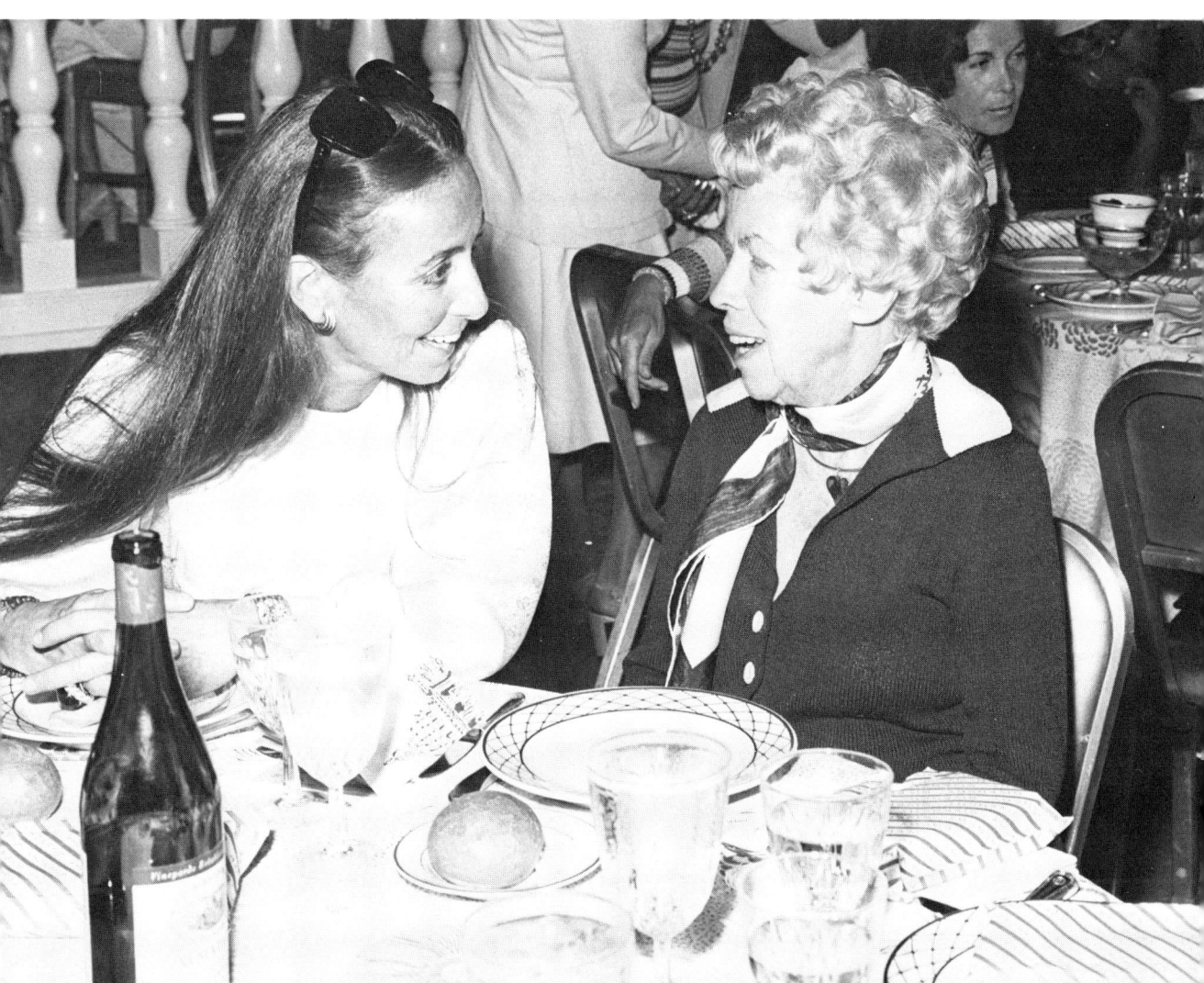

floor, or their eyes are in constant motion, scanning the room and everyone in it. This can be disconcerting. I'm distinctly uncomfortable talking to people who won't look me in the eye. It's like trying to carry on a conversation with the little man who wasn't there. It also makes me wonder what they're hiding, what they know that they don't want me to know. It's not a pleasant feeling. It makes me feel that if they had a magazine or newspaper, they'd hold it in front of their faces.

If you're not in the habit of making eye contact with people, start practicing right now. Yes, you may feel a little uncomfortable about it at first, but I promise you, it will get easier as you go along. And here's another thing: even in those situations where you feel less than perfectly confident and at ease, no one will guess it if you're able to make and hold eye contact with each person in the room.

SMALL TALK: Most social talk *is* small talk. I don't know whether that is good or bad. It's just a fact.

Unfortunately, a lot of people haven't grasped the fact. They're the ones who automatically clam up when they think they're out of their depth either socially or intellectually. They're under the impression that if they're going to talk to certain people at all, it has to be brilliant, or amusing, or meaningful, serious talk and they doubt their ability to carry it off. They needn't feel that way.

My friend Louis Nizer and I don't talk law at a dinner party. We usually ramble on about current events and art. People don't want to talk about what they do all day. They want to relax.

Granted, some people are better at small talk than others. (In fact, some people are so good at it that they rattle on and on forever about the weather, their pets, or whatever, and the problem then is how to turn them off. We'll get to that one later.) But anyone can become reasonably adept at it.

To begin with, there are three or four topics that practically guarantee at least five minutes of successful small talk each. Don't hesitate to use them.

One is the joy and/or heartbreak of parenting. Anyone with kids loves to talk about them. It's just as true of Cheray and Peter Duchin as it is the stay-at-home wife and mother. (Maybe more so.)

Incidentally, most of the grandparents I know would rather talk about their grandchildren than their children.

Sure-fire topic number two is food—and not just for women, but for men, too. That's because most people these days are either dieting and get a vicarious thrill out of talk about all the things they *can't* eat, or they're in the process of discovering the joys of gourmet cooking. Obviously, if you're at a party or dinner, it's easy to get this kind of small talk going. You simply comment on the food being served. (Food talk almost always leads to restaurant talk, which is another sure-fire topic. *Everyone* has two or three favorite restaurants they want to tell you about. Everyone also takes pleasure in knocking—and warning everybody else away from—the high-priced status-y restaurant where the service was slow and snippy and the food abominable.)

Another good topic is "What are things coming to?" This is probably the easiest one of all to introduce. All you have to do is mention the horrendous traffic jam you got stuck in on the way over, or the cost of coffee, or the pornography displayed on all the newsstands, and you're off and running.

Doctors—how to find a good internist, who's the best allergist in town, that sort of thing—are a favorite topic of almost everyone who isn't a doctor, but it's not always an easy one to introduce. (Someone has to sneeze or complain of a headache before you can really get into it.)

California is another good one. Hardly anyone is neutral on the subject. Most people either love it or loathe it, or they love one part of it and loathe the other, and they want to tell you exactly why they feel the way they do. Especially if you're from New York.

Finally, an old dull opening gambit—"You're looking *wonderful* lately"—is beginning to yield some amazingly good results as a small-talk starter. That's because suddenly almost everyone has become so conscious of physical fitness. Chances are if someone you know really *is* looking better than ever, it's because he or she has taken up jogging or tennis or Yoga. If so, that person will want to tell you all about it. (Of course, that marvelous, well-rested new look could be the result of a face-lift, or silicone treatments, or the start of a love affair. In

which case, the response to "You're looking wonderful" will probably be a simple dead-end "Thank you, you're looking well yourself."
SMALL TALK TO AVOID: Small talk by definition is light, amiable, a pleasant way to establish contact with new people and keep in touch with old acquaintances. The idea, as in any kind of talk, is to communicate your thoughts, your feelings, your opinions—and if you have a way with a wry, witty anecdote, so much the better. No subject is taboo. You can make small talk about sex, or astrophysics, or even politics for that matter (though when the interchange becomes heated or technical or very personal, you've left the realm of small talk and moved on to something else). But there are some kinds of small talk that I always try to stay away from.

"Girl talk" is one of them. It's lovely to give and receive compliments. When another woman tells me she likes my dress, I'm always very pleased and I thank her. But if she goes on from there to ask me who designed it, have I seen the new Valentino collection in the latest *Vogue*, and what do I think of the blouson look, I know I'm in trouble. She wants to talk girl talk.

It's not that I *never* want to discuss clothes and designers and makeup and hairdressers. Like most women, I enjoy it—but only once in a while, and usually when I'm on the phone, or visiting with a friend. I'm extremely reluctant to get involved in girl talk in a male/female social situation, mainly because of the way it divides the men from the women. (Haven't you ever been to a party where all the women were planted in chairs on one side of the room talking about clothes and all the men on the other side talking business and sports? And after a while, wasn't it a crashing bore?) My feeling about small talk is that it should be a game *anyone* can play.

Shoptalk between people who work together or who are involved in the same kind of professional activity is almost as bad as girl talk and I dislike it for the same reason: it excludes others—in the case of shoptalk, anyone who isn't intimately acquainted with the details of the business can't join in. Actually, shoptalk isn't small talk at all since it tends to be so technical and "weighty." Telling people about the kind of work you do and why you like it and how you got into it is something else again. It's small talk and it can be fascinating.

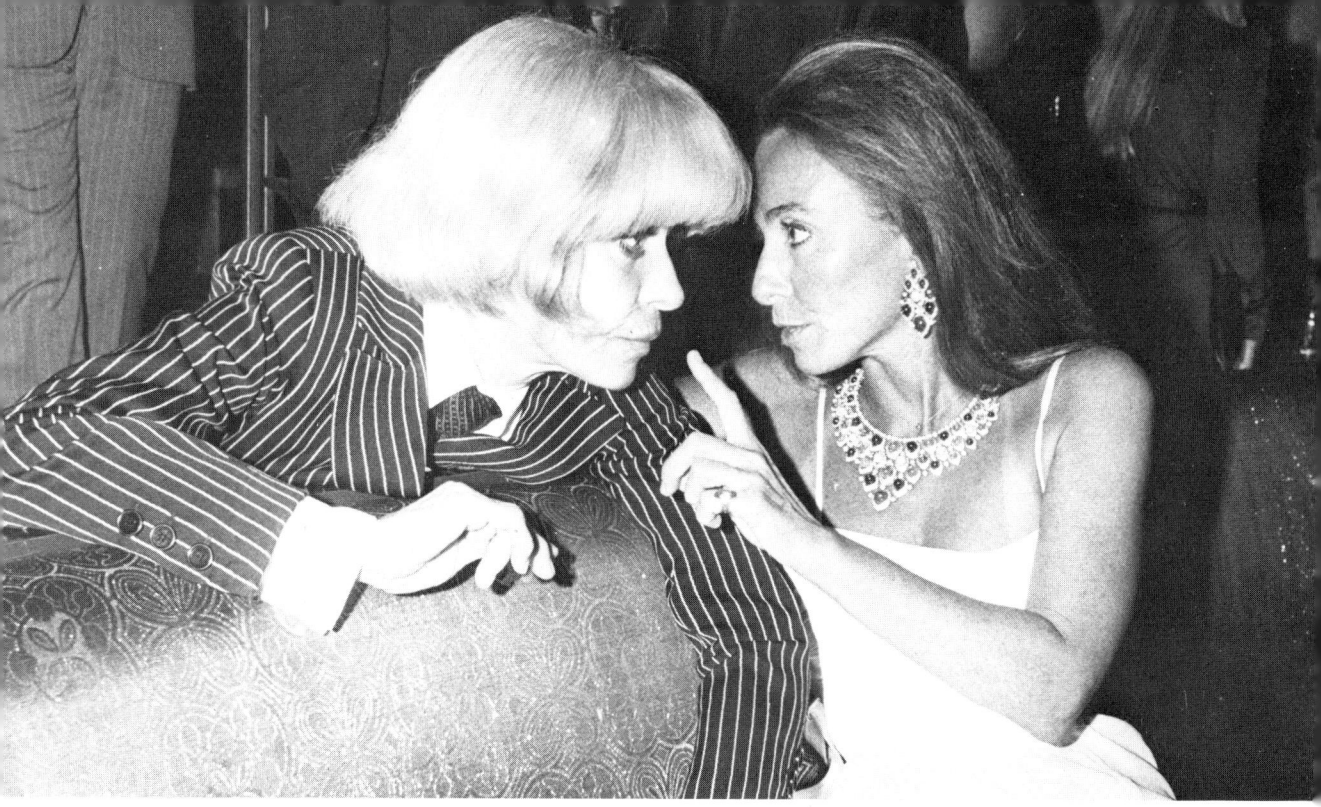

At a dinner party given by Carol Channing at Regine's. (PHOTO: NEW YORK *Post*)

As for asking someone outright "What do you do?", I think it's an offensive kind of inquiry. At least I've always felt that way about it. The question is hardly ever asked out of innocent curiosity. Instead, it's usually used as a device to gauge status, for "placing" people with regard to how much money or power they have, or their social standing. The kind of person who asks "What do you do?" is apt to dismiss as not worth bothering about anyone who isn't involved in important, high-status work. (These people may be interested to know that anyone who does important, high-status work is apt to dismiss the person who asks "What do you do?" as a boor.)

Whenever I'm confronted with this particular question, I'm always tempted to answer, "As well as I can, thank you." And then move away as quickly as possible.

Gossiping is another kind of small talk that I generally avoid. I don't mean to say that I don't gossip at all; *everyone* does it once in a while. But I don't do it at parties or in other social situations, and

I never do it with people I don't know well. It's too risky. It's impossible to predict what the consequences of gossiping with a stranger might be.

I remember once chatting with a man I'd just met at a party. He mentioned the name of another guest, a woman, who was standing several feet away with a small group of people. He glanced over in her direction, lowered his voice, and then proceeded to tell me a long, involved story in which she came off *very* badly. Halfway through the story, I interrupted him to say that the woman in question happened to be a very good friend of mine, that he had the story all wrong, and that I hoped he wouldn't repeat it to anyone else. Genuinely embarrassed, he apologized and assured me he would stop telling the story. I run into him from time to time and he *still* seems uncomfortable about the incident. That's fine with me.

Asking about someone's divorce is never a good idea. Worse still is to ask when there are three or four other people standing idly by. (And asking anything whatsoever about the financial settlement is practically unforgivable.) Even the most widely publicized divorce is an intensely private matter. If a woman in the throes of getting unmarried wants to tell you about it, she will. (This is true for men, too, of course.) But if she doesn't bring it up, there's no reason for anyone else to refer to it.

Serious illness, death in the family, financial catastrophe, loss of a job—all are best treated in the same way as divorce. If you want to express your concern to the person with major problems, then by all means put on a sympathetic expression and ask how he or she is doing. You'll get your message across. If the person responds with a simple "Thank you, I'm getting by all right," then leave it at that.

If you're a sensitive, tactful person yourself, I can understand how these cautionary words might seem entirely unnecessary. But believe me, there are people—some of them with impeccable social credentials—who don't hesitate to pry in the most obvious, offensive way into the personal affairs of others. I won't name names but I've seen it happen many times and it's a painful thing to watch. So I excuse myself and go off to join another group.

How to Know if You're a Bore and What to Do About It

An old, old friend once said, "Call me a bitch, call me a loudmouth, call me a dumb broad, but don't call me a bore." I think she did a pretty good job of summing it up for the rest of us. Most people would rather be thought of as *anything* but boring. Yet, the world continues to be overrun by bores (granted, some of them are boring only some of the time), and I think we have to conclude from that that when people are being boring, they don't know it. Which leads to a rather unsettling thought: if "people" can be boring without being aware of it, so could *I*. Or *you*. Or anyone.

Except that I believe it's possible to avoid being a bore simply by making a conscious effort to avoid doing things that are boring.

What's boring?

Talking on and on about oneself definitely qualifies. This is unfortunate because we are, each of us, our own favorite, most fascinating topic of conversation—a subject none of us can ever exhaust. No matter who we happen to be, however, it's entirely possible to exhaust our listeners. And it usually happens sooner rather than later. Keep it in mind next time you're at a social gathering and feel the temptation to unreel your life story from beginning to end. Only a mother or a lover wants to know every last little detail, and as a person who has had experience as both, I'm not sure that even mothers and lovers are all *that* much interested.

If talking too much about oneself is boring, and it is, so is talking about oneself in certain *ways*. If the point of all your stories is to illustrate how unfair or unkind people and fate have been to you, perhaps you'd better change the endings or get some new stories. Painting oneself as the eternal victim is a bore.

So is being the eternal heroine of every anecdote you tell. (I know a woman who, to judge from her conversation, has never made an error in judgment, never lost an argument, never lacked the insight to come up with the solution to other people's problems, and never failed to deal successfully with her own. She is the most tedious person imaginable.)

Enumerating one's possessions is boring. It becomes positively irritating when prices and manufacturers' or designers' names are included with the listing.

Complaints are boring. Especially complaints about the weather, the servants, minor health problems, putting on weight, and the town you live in.

Unless you're a crackerjack storyteller, most jokes are boring too. So is trying too hard to be funny. But the straight, stony-faced approach can be just as bad, and speaking in a dull, droning monotone has a decidedly soporific effect. (No, we can't all be witty, polished raconteurs, but we can all put a little more verve in our talk by varying facial expressions and tone of voice to go with the stories.)

Certain mannerisms can be so distracting that in self-defense people have to turn off to them. Boredom is the inevitable result. I'm thinking of things like fidgeting in one's chair, tapping a pencil on a tabletop, nervous giggling or clearing of the throat. The woman who constantly smooths her hair or who is always digging deep into her bag for a mirror to inspect her makeup is ultimately boring. So is the man who straightens his tie every few seconds.

The person who carries on a conversation while his eyes go darting about the room, watching for new arrivals and checking to see who's talking to whom, is a bore. In fact, anyone whose attention is obviously focused elsewhere is boring to talk to (which reminds me of a certain prominent jeweler who never makes eye contact because he's always so busy evaluating your earrings, your bracelets, your watch).

If you think you recognize anything of yourself in the last few paragraphs, don't despair. You're not doomed to be a bore forever. You can change. You're taking a big first step simply by becoming more aware of how boring certain kinds of talk and modes of expression can be. The next step is to try not to repeat yourself in the future.

As far as I'm concerned, the biggest bore of all is the bored person. Unfortunately, pulling yourself up out of your boredom is no easy accomplishment. People with money spend thousands, sometimes millions of dollars on clothing, travel, cars, yachts, beach houses, racehorses, and other grown-up toys in the effort to alleviate their boredom. But boredom isn't the exclusive privilege of the very rich. People with little money get bored too and try to work out other, less expensive solutions to their problems.

I don't think anything you can buy—with the possible exception of time spent with a psychotherapist—cures boredom. The cure, if there is one, comes from within, from a certain enthusiasm for life and people and the things around one. Everyone is born with it. Some people keep it forever. Others lose it fairly early on. Nobody knows exactly how or why. It's very sad.

How to Deal with a Bore

Over the last few years I've made it my policy never to invite to my home anyone whose company I don't enjoy. I haven't the time or the patience to tolerate tedious, uninteresting people, and I'm fortunate because my life is arranged in such a way that I don't need to.

The bores one meets at a party, at a gallery opening, in the lobby of a theater, at a fund-raising dinner—that's something else again. Dealing with them requires special strategies. I'm not entirely satisfied with the set of strategies I've developed, but I'll pass them along to you for whatever they're worth. (If you can think of any better ones, please write me care of my publisher.)

1. Avoidance. I've never gone so far as to hide behind someone's potted palm to escape the notice of a notorious bore, but I have skipped off to the ladies' room when I saw one headed my way. (Usually, I give a little wave of the hand as I pass by.) This strategy works with known bores, but for obvious reasons it's useless when it suddenly hits you that the man your hostess has just introduced to you is going to go on talking all evening about his Siamese cats if you don't do something about it. In such situations, strategies 2 or 3 may be helpful.

2. Get hungry or thirsty. This one only works if there's a bar or

table across the room where refreshments are being served. (It doesn't work at all if there are waiters circulating with trays of champagne and hors d'oeuvres, or if you're seated at the dinner table.) To carry it off, you have to say something like, "I'm terribly sorry to interrupt, but I think I'll perish right here on the spot if I don't get something to eat [or drink]. Excuse me for just a minute, please." Then you hurry off in search of food [or drink]. If you're lucky, you'll bump into an old friend on the way and become so absorbed in this new conversation that you'll "forget" all about returning to the bore.

3. Change the subject. This is practically the only way to deal with boring talk when you're trapped at the dinner table and can't get away. When the person you're seated next to launches into what promises to be a long-winded lecture on a topic in which you're not the slightest bit interested, you may be able to divert him or her by saying something like, "Excuse me, but what you just said reminds me of a line from the new Robert Altman film. Have you seen it?" No, this isn't polite, but it allows you to get a word in edgewise and in the process to gain control of the conversation and get it going in a direction that is more enjoyable to you.

4. Introduce a friend. This one is really much kinder to the bore than strategies 1, 2, and 3, but it may be a little hard on your friend. When you realize you've got a bore on your hands, you look around for someone you know, then say to the bore, "Excuse me, there's someone I want you to meet." Walk over to your friend and drag him or her back with you to the bore, then introduce them. At this point you can do one of two things. You can start up a long, intense conversation with your friend, leaving the bore out of it. Or you can suddenly get hungry or thirsty and leave your friend to deal with the bore.

What to Do about a Boring Friend

Do you have a friend (or husband or someone else who is close to you) who every once in a while tends to get stuck on a particular topic and goes on and on about it over and over again like a broken record? Well, I do. Her thing is a certain charity. She is passionately involved with this charity, gives it many, many hours of her time, and that's good. What isn't good is that she brings her enthusiasm with her to parties and other social gatherings, where she invariably gets up on her soapbox (figuratively) and begins an emotional appeal to others on behalf of her cause. After a few minutes of this she becomes a bore.

I'm fond of her and I hate to see others turning off to her, as they eventually do. I especially hate to see others turning off to her when the party is at *my* house, because then I feel a special responsibility to keep things lively and not let the conversation get bogged down.

So I try to step in and shut her up, to save her from herself and to save my party as well.

It isn't easy. It has to be done in a way that isn't obvious to the other guests and at the same time doesn't hurt or offend my friend. To pull it off, I have to wait until she pauses for breath and then quickly leap in with a question that has nothing to do with fund-raising and charities—preferably a question that will not only divert the conversation to another topic, but one that will make my friend feel good as well. Such as, "Mary [not her real name], I wanted to ask you before I forget, what was the name of that artist who did the marvelous painting in your bedroom?"

If I can't think of an appropriate question for Mary, then I try to toss in a comment directed specifically to one of the other guests—a comment that is vaguely related to what Mary has been saying, but not so closely that she can respond to it herself (and thereby catch the conversational ball and run off with it again). For example, if Mary has been talking about raising funds for her project I might ask one of the other guests about the progress of the charity ball *he's* been working on. That sort of thing.

Occasionally, I've had to resort to more involved maneuverings. Like excusing myself, going back to the kitchen, and asking the cook if she can *please* hurry dinner along. (Any change of scene—in this case, a move to the dining room—presents opportunities for new conversational openings.) Or, if it's a Sunday night and I'm doing the cooking, I'll suddenly remember I have to make some last-minute preparations and invite anyone who wants to to come back to the kitchen to keep me company. Once I even jumped up and asked everyone to come see the new baby fish that had just hatched in the tank in my dressing room.

Desperate measures. But sometimes they need to be taken to save a friend and a party.

When You Go as a Couple

When married people leave the house for a social evening, they do themselves and everyone else a favor by leaving their problems at their own doorstep. Of course, we all want to lend sympathetic and understanding ears to couples with problems who are our friends. But there's a time and a place for everything.

I can't think of many situations more strained and uncomfortable than being in the company of a husband and wife who snipe endlessly back and forth at each other across the dinner table. Almost as bad as when husband and wife are pointedly speaking to everyone else but not one another. Under the circumstances, sympathy disappears. Old friends or not, one only wishes that the warring couple had stayed at home.

One couple I know assumed that their bickering was *amusing*. The wife said as much one day when she referred to the way she and her husband had "livened up the party" the night before. Apparently, they hadn't noticed the desperate expression on the face of the hostess as she struggled valiantly to divert the pair and maneuver them to opposite sides of the room.

Airing private concerns in someone else's dining room or living room isn't amusing. It's selfish and inconsiderate because of the strain it imposes on hostess and guests alike.

And then there are the happy lovebirds who stay pasted together from the minute they arrive to the time they leave. It's nice to see couples who are fond of each other. But when a husband and wife form an exclusive little group of two, when they're so totally absorbed in one another that they hardly seem to be aware of the other guests, they aren't very interesting and they're certainly not contributing to the party.

(Actually, I'm always suspicious when I see a couple *that* wrapped up in each other. Often, there's something other than total love and devotion going on—something like jealousy or fear or insecurity on the part of one of them, who simply won't *allow* the other to talk to, or even look at, anyone else. It reminds me of the woman who at parties becomes permanently attached to the arm of her husband—"the pussycat," she calls him. The pussycat is *such* a pussycat that, according to her, he never, ever gripes or complains and life at their house is just a bed of roses. Which all leads me to wonder whether his gripes and complaints—he *must* have them, everyone does—aren't all being heard by someone else. Who maybe calls him "tiger"?)

One more thing: husbands and wives, as every married person knows, aren't always in perfect sync about their social lives. Some wives would like nothing better than to go out every night of the week, while what their husbands really want to do is come home from work, unwind, have a quiet private dinner, and then fall into bed at nine o'clock. (Of course, it isn't always the wife who wants to go out every night; sometimes it's the other way around.)

It can get to be a problem, a big one.

When husbands and wives have different social needs or desires, each partner has to give a little. It helps to remember that a marriage with *no* social input almost always becomes dull, stultifying. But spending no time at home alone together can make a couple feel like strangers to one another. That's no good either. Compromising somewhere in the middle makes more sense.

Finally, to the spouse whose mate sits through a social evening with all the enthusiasm and animation of a corpse, try to understand why—instead of attacking the minute you reach home.

He or she may have been just too bone tired to do anything else.

How to Handle the Marijuana Question

It's bound to happen. Sooner or later someone will offer you marijuana. If you're already a smoker and enjoy it, there's no problem. If you don't smoke it and don't want to, there's still no problem. Simply shake your head and say, "No, thanks," just as you would if someone had offered you a cigarette or drink you didn't want.

Many women who have no qualms about turning down a cigarette or drink are reluctant to pass up marijuana because they're afraid to be thought "out of it." Or they think that to refuse marijuana is somehow to pass a negative judgment on the people who do use it.

It's always a mistake to do something you don't particularly want to do just because "everyone" else is doing it, or because you're worried about what others will think if you don't do it. That's just as true of smoking marijuana as it is of anything else.

The Evening that Never Gets Off the Ground

We've all spent social evenings that never got off the ground. Sometimes an evening flops despite the fact that all the ingredients for success are in evidence: good food, a lovely setting, a roomful of dynamic, interesting, attractive people.

I spent an evening like that several months ago. It was truly memorable for its lack of success. There were eight people present. The men were the kind best described as "high-powered." The women were all active, busy, creative people though there were very few careerists among them. In any event, I think you would be familiar with the names of perhaps six out of the eight people in that room.

My escort and I were seated at a table for eight. Among those at the table were an oil executive, a theatrical producer, and a financier. Only a few necessary introductions were made because many of the people already knew one another. I turned to the man at my right and asked him about something we'd discussed the last time we met. My escort, a genial, intelligent man who could charm a stone if he had to, opened a conversation with the woman at his left.

I realized as the soup was being served that no one else was talking. Aside from our four voices, there was only the clink, clink, clink of silver against china. I caught my escort's eye. He shrugged very slightly and then called out something to a woman across the table from him. I in turn leaned over and made a remark to a man seated off to my left. Now there was a new quartet of voices, but everyone else was silent. Feeling a little desperate and talking to everyone in general and no one in particular, I began to tell a story about something that had happened to me the day before—not the most amusing story, I must admit, but one that anyone present could have picked up on and gone somewhere with. When I finished, there were one or two murmurs. Then more silence.

I gave up after that and so did my escort. I'd tried my best and so had he. It was simply one of those evenings.

I've tried to figure out *why* it sometimes happens that a whole group of people who've gathered together for a social evening can't bring themselves to be sociable. It's a mystery. The best explanation I can come up with for this particular disaster was that it happened on a Friday night. Maybe by sheer coincidence everyone present had had an especially hectic and tiring week. Maybe they were all half asleep in their chairs. Who knows?

The point is that these evenings do happen. They're difficult to get through but they're not the end of the world. If you happen to be the unlucky hostess of one of these parties, don't beat yourself. It's not your fault, your guests will survive and so will you. And if you happen to be one of the guests, don't pity the poor hostess. It happens to the best of them.

How and When to Leave

A hostess will almost always be specific about when the party begins but often leaves the question of when it's over to her guests—assuming, I suppose, that they'll all have the good sense to go home at a reasonable hour. Well, sometimes they do and sometimes they don't, as anyone who entertains frequently knows. I'm sure that no one purposely overstays his or her welcome. It's just that there are sometimes doubts about the reasonable hour for leaving. (I know that many people fear being considered "impolite" if they leave too early, so they end up staying far too late.)

For me and most of the people I know, sometime between ten thirty and eleven thirty is a "reasonable" time to leave almost any kind of social gathering during the week. That's because most of the men, if not the women, have to be up and at work fairly early the next morning. If you're ready to leave at eleven but the party is still going strong and all of the other guests look as though they're going to camp there till morning, what do you do?

Very simple: you approach the hostess, tell her it's been a lovely evening, say good-bye to her and anyone else you want to say good-bye to, and leave. What if your host and hostess give you a hard time about leaving, urging you to stay a while longer, pointing out that the party's hardly begun? Then stay if you want to. If not, it's perfectly okay to explain to them that you and/or your husband or escort have to be up early the next day and really *must* leave. Then leave.

(Incidentally, if it's a *very* large party with more than fifty or sixty guests, I don't believe it's absolutely necessary to elbow your way through the crowd in order to say good-night to your host and hostess, especially if you're among the very first to leave. In fact, it's probably better to slip out quietly and then phone or send a note the following day, thanking them for the very pleasant evening.)

At a dinner party, you don't need to stay any longer than, say, ten or fifteen minutes after coffee has been served. Stay longer, of course, if you want to. But you needn't feel that you must.

People often want to stay out later on Friday and Saturday nights and the host and hostess may expect their guests to linger on till one or two o'clock. Even then, there's no reason to feel you must stay longer than ten to fifteen minutes after coffee if you're tired or just want to go home.

I think the best time to leave a party, whether it's a week-night or weekend event, is just after it peaks. (I'm sure you've noticed many times that most parties have a little "life cycle" of their own: guests arrive, introductions are made, conversational groups form, break up, and re-form, people feel more and more relaxed and at ease, there's a crescendo of talk and laughter, then it all starts to run down. You can almost tell the peak by the noise level.) Where parties are concerned, "always leave them laughing" is a good motto.

Certainly, when the host and hostess stop looking attentive and start exchanging meaningful glances, when their smiles begin to look pasted on and their eyes glaze over, it's time to get going. It was time to leave half an hour ago! If you've somehow stayed on till that point, you would be doing your host and hostess a great kindness if you could somehow find a way to alert the other stragglers that the party is indeed over.

Special Gifts for Special People

No one—but no one—is so blasé that the arrival of a package imaginatively wrapped, obviously a present, doesn't stir a little thrill of anticipation. *Everyone* loves a gift. That's why gift-giving is such a nice style to cultivate.

"JUST BECAUSE" GIFTS: "I'm not just thinking about the big-occasion gift—the birthday gift, the anniversary gift, the holiday gift. Those gifts are important and fun to get, of course. But they're also usually expected. Even required. No, what I have in mind is the marvelously thoughtful and personal expression of your feelings represented by the kind of gift you give "just because." Just because you like someone or miss someone or think you might

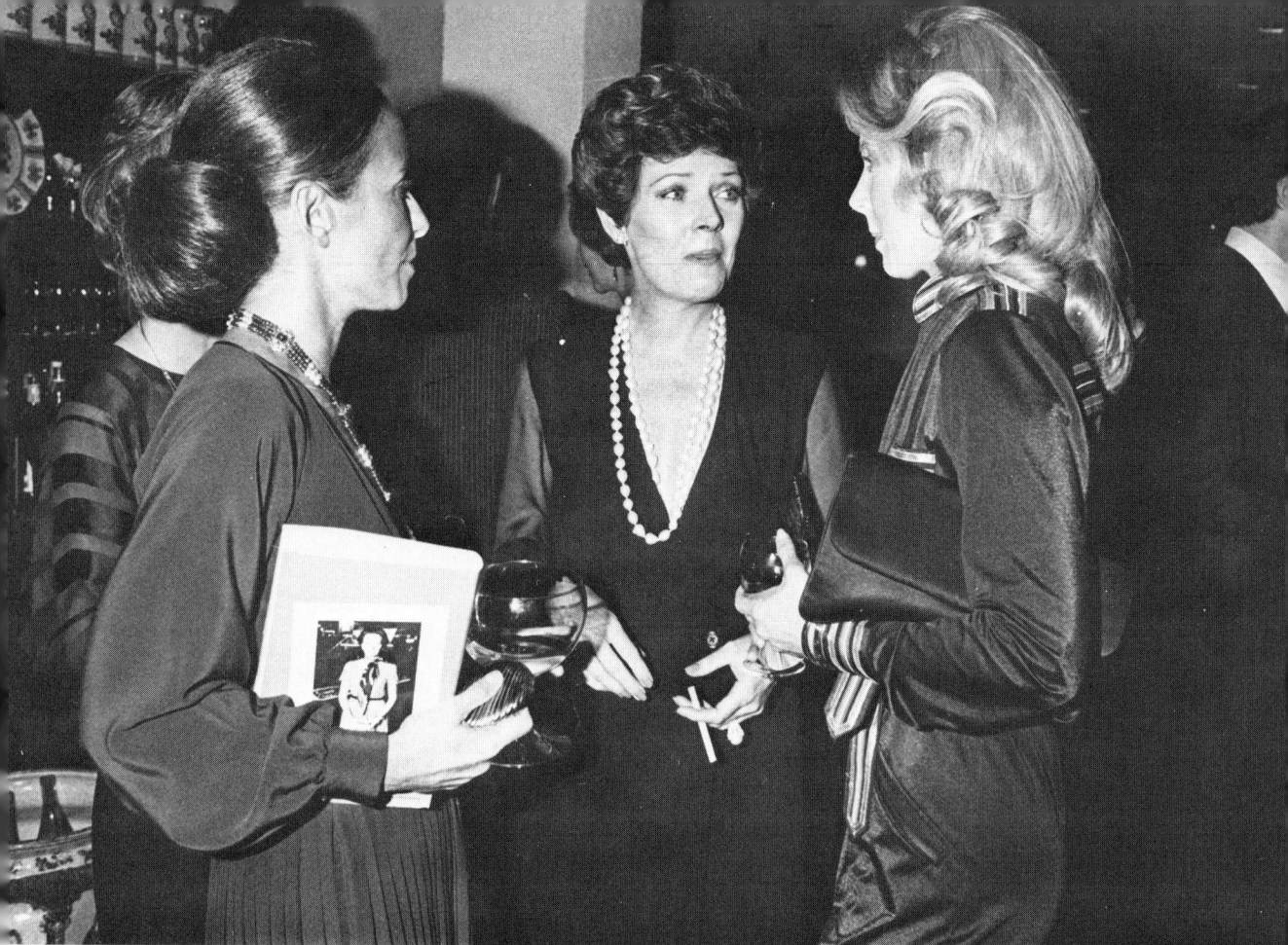

With Polly Bergen and my good friend Joan Schnitzer at a cocktail reception in honor of writer and editor Charlotte Curtis. (PHOTO: ABNER SYMONS/WWD)

want to know someone better. Just because you had a wonderful time at a party and you want to make sure the host and hostess know it. Just because you've heard about someone's promotion or new business venture and you want to say how pleased you are about it. Just because you want to show your appreciation for something someone's done for you.

I know that a phone call would do in any of these cases, and it's certainly easier to pick up the telephone and simply *say* what you're feeling. But that's just the point. Selecting a gift and having it wrapped and delivered requires that you go a little bit out of your way: it *means* more.

"Just because" gifts needn't cost a lot of money. Indeed, they shouldn't. A present that you've obviously spent a bundle on is fine for a husband or lover, son or daughter, mother, father, or very close friend. But buying an expensive gift for someone "just because" can make the recipient feel extremely uncomfortable. He or she may wonder about your motives, what you're "angling for" in return for the gift, or may feel vaguely "obligated" (which is never pleasant).

Besides, anyone can go to Tiffany or Neiman-Marcus or some other fabulous store and pick out a present to make the eyes pop. Giving an extravagant "just because" gift isn't necessarily an expression of great style. More likely, it's mere ostentatious spending, which doesn't say much about you except that you've got a lot of money to throw around—or that you don't handle the money you do have very wisely.

The ideal "just because" gift says only good things about you. That you're generous. Warm. A person of imagination and taste who has a knack for always choosing just the right thing.

What kind of gift items fill the bill? Well, there are so many different kinds that it's hard to know just where to begin, but I'll start out with some of the "just because" gifts that have made a special impression on me.

A small potted flowering cactus. To the plant lover, almost any small plant makes a marvelous gift. Incidentally, a very special way to give a plant is in a "personalized" clay pot. I get these at Mädderlake florist on Madison Avenue. (I assume they write the name in the clay before it dries; when it hardens, the name is there for good.)

A bundle of felt-tipped marking pens, all different colors, tied with a ribbon.

A big glass jar filled all the way to the top with jelly beans or licorice or candy kisses.

Dried flowers in a scented straw basket.

Straw baskets of any size or shape, from the largest ones that are big enough to hold firewood or magazines to very small ones in the shape of animals. (The latter can be used to hold nuts or candy and the ones I've seen at Plumbridge on Madison Avenue in New York are decorative enough to have a permanent place on a mantel or table.)

Four or five note pads, each in a different vivid color. These make nice Christmas gifts, too, if you order them in time to have the recipient's name or initials put on them.

A coffee mug or pair of mugs printed with the recipient's first name or initial. (These don't need to be ordered in advance. Many department stores have a selection of preprinted mugs.)

A dozen tennis balls or golf balls. (Obviously, for the person or couple who plays tennis or golf.)

Scented candles.

Two pounds of cashews or other nuts. See if you can get a big burlap sack to put them in; tie shut with heavy twine. I get the best unsalted ones at Perrone's on Third Avenue.

A box of good chocolates. (Kron's on Madison Avenue in New York will put a chocolate card in a wooden box, made like a packing crate, with a specially printed message on the chocolate. Tell them the message you want on the card—"Thanks for the use of your tennis court," "Terrific party"—and have them send it along. Another Kron's specialty is a box made of chocolate with chocolate candies inside. For a laugh, they'll make up chocolate sculptures. Someone I know sent someone else a chocolate sculptured woman's leg. That sort of thing.)

A cookbook. (If one of your dinner guests asks about one of the dishes you've served, why not send along the cookbook that contains the recipe?)

A bundle of wooden cooking utensils in a small wooden keg, or tied with a ribbon.

A good French omelette pan.

A special accessory or part for a Cuisinart or other cooking machine. (But only if the person already owns the machine itself, of course.)

Cocktail napkins. Very special if they're from Porthault.

Games. People, at least the people I know, are definitely playing more games lately. Monopoly, Thought Wave, Risk, Scrabble, all are good choices. So are many of the other grown-up games available in many department stores and bookshops such as Brentano's. Backgammon and chess sets are nice, too, but the good ones are usually priced too high for the "just because" gift category. Save them for birthdays or anniversaries instead.

A poster, especially the kind that announces the opening of a major museum exhibition. Art posters are good, too. Look for them in museum gift shops. (Many museum gift shops are treasure troves of the kind of attractive, moderately priced gifts we're talking about here. In New York, the Metropolitan Museum of Art and the Brooklyn Museum are particularly good sources.)

A bottle or two of good wine.

A sampler of different kinds of tea or coffee. Or a pound or two of the recipient's favorite tea or coffee. (Obviously, I'm not talking about Lipton's and Maxwell House now, but the kind that comes from a fine specialty shop or from the gourmet food department of a good department store.)

A jar or two of English marmalade or jam. (Even nicer, marmalade or jam that you've made and labeled yourself.)

A whole wheel of a favorite cheese.

A small jar of caviar.

A small jar of black licorice candy that looks exactly like caviar.

A best-selling book—one you know that the recipient has been dying to read (or one on a subject that is of particular interest to him or her).

A record. Popular, classical, Broadway show music, or whatever is in line with the recipient's musical tastes.

A shiny metal, clear Lucite, or other moderately priced but good-looking picture frame (no one ever has enough of them). Better still if it holds a blown-up snapshot of the recipient taken on some occasion when you and she or he were together.

Six or eight wine glasses. Or iced tea glasses or good-looking tumblers.

A scented pillow. Porthault has some very pretty ones with different scents and different sayings embroidered across them.

A subscription to *Vogue, Bazaar, House & Garden, Architectural Digest, The New Yorker, Gourmet* magazine, or any magazine you know the recipient enjoys reading.

HOUSE GIFTS AND THANK-YOU GIFTS: Almost all the items mentioned so far make wonderful thank-you gifts, the kind you really *must* send after spending a weekend as a guest at someone's home, or to someone who has done something especially nice for you (such as sponsoring you for club membership, or introducing you or your husband to a person who later becomes a big client).

BIRTHDAY, CHRISTMAS, AND ANNIVERSARY GIFTS: Many of the items just mentioned are also perfect as birthday, Christmas, and anniversary gifts for the people in the "middle distance" of your life—by which I mean the people you work with or who work for you and all but your very closest friends and relatives. (Not included in this group are the doormen, elevator operators, and superintendents of your apartment building, your maid if you have one, your hairdresser and manicurist, your doctor's and dentist's receptionists. All of these people are in a different gift-giving category, and we'll get to them later.)

A marvelous anniversary gift to consider, especially if the couple have lived together happily for a long time, is wine or cognac bottled in the year of their marriage. Or, for a birthday, wine or cognac bottled in the year of the recipient's birth.

Another tip for anniversary gifts: you can always take your cue from the number of years the couple have been married. A second anniversary, for example, is the "cotton" anniversary. So, for the cotton anniversary of former Mayor and Mrs. Robert Wagner, a friend and I bought giant-size Raggedy Ann and Andy dolls (because they're made of cotton). Fastened securely to one of Andy's hands was a bottle of Dom Perignon champagne. Ann held two Baccarat wine glasses in her hands, and we tucked a Porthault cocktail napkin into each pocket of her pinafore.

The handmade present is *always* very meaningful. The knitted sweater, the crocheted afghan take time, which is for many people

Friends and Other People / 137

more precious than money. Thus, the gift has an ultraspecial meaning both to the giver and the receiver. I love to do needlepoint, and when I have time, I make gifts (usually pillows, sometimes a whole rug) for the very important people in my life.

Don't overlook the gag present for people who enjoy that kind of thing. Not long ago, a group of people got together on a present for Bill Fine, president of Frances Denney Cosmetics. We took a huge, heavyweight plastic garbage bag and filled it with a 9 1/2-foot bag of

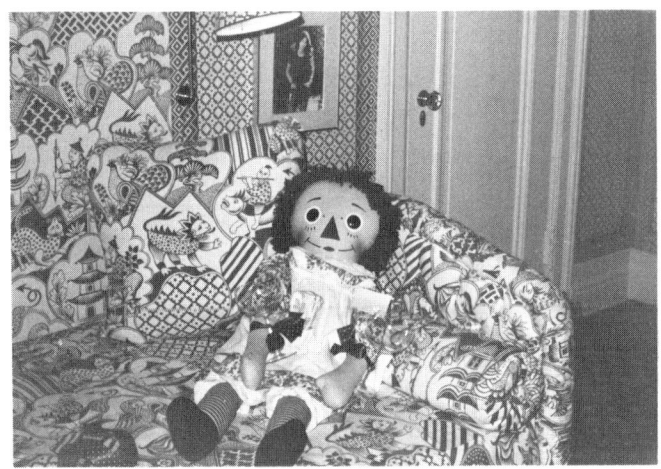

A "cotton" (second) anniversary gift for Mr. and Mrs. Robert Wagner: huge Raggedy Ann and Andy dolls. Here's Ann, a wine goblet in each hand, Porthault cocktail napkins tucked in her pockets; Andy holds champagne. (PHOTO: LYN REVSON)

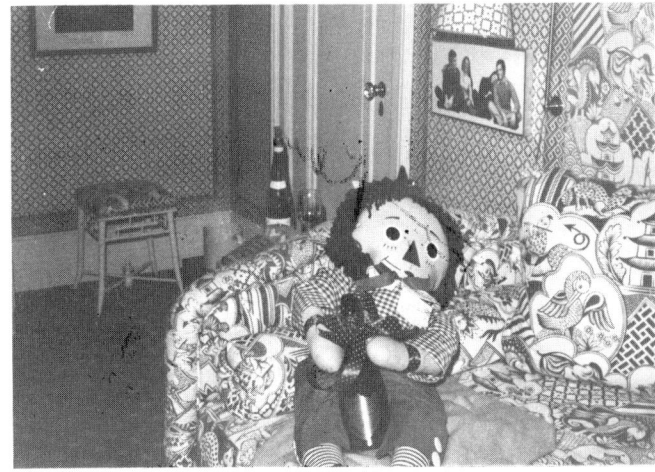

popcorn. We threw in a tie, a couple of pairs of shoe-socks (really socks with plastic soles, the kind children sometimes wear as bedroom slippers) with track shoes printed on the sock part, a bottle of cologne, a belt, a box of four tiny shot glasses shaped like mugs (these were packaged in a little box that said "Mug Shots" on it). Then we tied it all together with a ribbon and a flower and a sack of soap with $1,000,000 printed on it.

GIFTS TO AVOID: Very personal items such as perfume, cologne or toiletries, jewelry, lingerie, and almost any gift meant to be worn should be saved for the people you know quite well. First, because unless you know for sure the person's preference in these items and/or their size, it's awfully easy to make a mistake. And the gift that has to be returned or exchanged is a nuisance. Also, there are still some people to whom a personal gift from a woman to a man, or from a man to a woman, implies a sexual interest. (Actually, I think very few people feel that way anymore, but some do. Keep it in mind. Naturally, if your interest *is* sexual, by all means give an intimate gift.)

An expensive gift from a store that won't accept merchandise for exchange or refund usually isn't a good choice unless you're sure the person wants or can use the item. The same is true of the gift from a store which stocks only a very limited variety of merchandise. Here's a perfect example of why. Once I received a costly evening bag as a present. But I already have several evening bags, and, in fact, I'd rather *not* carry a bag at night and often go out without one. (I was surprised this particular person, whom I knew quite well, hadn't noticed this about me.) The store was quite willing to make an exchange, but evening bags were the only item of merchandise sold there. The result: the bag sat on a shelf for a long, long time until I finally gave it away. If at all possible, buy in a department store.

There's another little lesson in that story: the best gifts are always the ones that take personal preferences into account. The gift that overlooks those preferences often sets the recipient to wondering. Just what does it mean when someone you're close to sends you a gift which, if they know you at all, they know that you can't use or don't want? To me, it means someone else—a secretary perhaps—chose the gift. Or it means the person gave the same gift to everyone on his (or her) gift list. Or it may simply mean the person didn't give much thought to the gift. Sometimes, no gift at all is better than the thoughtless gift.

I'd also avoid hokey novelty-store items that are supposed to be amusing but aren't. I'm thinking now of things like those little books with "toilet jokes" in them, meant to be hung up in the bathroom for the amusement of guests, and other tacky, souvenir-type items.

By "hokey," I don't mean amusing or unusual or imaginative. (At the 1976 tennis matches in Forest Hills, I was bitten on the foot by a little bug called a blister beetle. It was no big thing, but my foot became very swollen and I had to stay off it for weeks. During that time a mysterious package arrived at my door. I unwrapped it and found an enormous wooden shoe, maybe two feet long, with a container inside filled with white roses. It was from Tony Martin and Cyd Charisse, and the card that came with it read, "If the shoe fits, go back to the doctor." It was fun to get and really *did* cheer me up.)

Gifts of cash or checks are inappropriate under most circumstances. They obviously don't belong to the "just because" category and to give cash or check on a birthday, Christmas, or anniversary—or even as a wedding present—is conspicuous evidence of taking the easy way out. I have a couple of friends who are top department store executives and they won't be happy to hear me say it, but the same is true of the department store gift certificate. Cash, checks, and gift certificates all imply that you didn't have the time or the imagination or the confidence in your own taste to give a real gift.

But there are a few instances where a gift certificate is a fine idea —especially if the certificate comes from a good store, one that has a superb reputation and a wide range of merchandise. A gift certificate from a boss to the secretary on her birthday is appropriate. A gift certificate is also a nice present for the person who does your hair or nails or walks your dog or cleans your house. Or for your doctor's or dentist's nurse or receptionist if she's been especially helpful about switching or juggling appointments.

As for the elevator operators, the doorman, the letter carrier, the superintendent of your building, and other people who make regular deliveries to your home, I may be wrong but I have the feeling that if you want to remember them at holiday time, a check is most appreciated.

How Not to Get Caught in the Christmas Crush

Jerome Zipkin, the best gift-giver I know, likes to brag about how he always has his Christmas shopping done by July (and usually adds "What's the matter with you, running around like a maniac the last week in December when anyone with any sense is sitting back taking it easy?").

Jerry's technique goes something like this: whenever he sees something that would make a good Christmas gift (usually because it reminds him of someone he knows), he buys it, no matter where he is or what time of year it happens to be. Then he makes a note of it, puts it away, and when Christmas comes, he wraps it and sends it off.

Jerry's way makes sense for a couple of reasons. There's the obvious one: he's not caught in the last-minute crunch. It also saves having to rack your brains for gift ideas at the very moment when the psychological pressure is greatest (and the ideas hardest to come by) and the supply of merchandise in the stores is rapidly dwindling. (I don't want to emphasize Jerry's efficiency at the expense of his creativity. He's an absolute genius at finding just the right gift—partly I suppose because he's always poking around in little out-of-the-way shops wherever he goes, and sees immediately the gift potential in the unusual, unique items he comes across.)

Wrappings That Say You

Just as a gift can be an expression of your personal style, so can the wrappings. (Of course you could have the store do your wrapping for you—Neiman-Marcus does the absolute best job of all—but then it becomes an expression of the *store's* style.)

For myself, I like the idea of choosing a "color scheme" each Christmas and using it for all the gifts I send out. One year it was heavy, shiny dark brown paper and olive green velvet ribbon. Another year it was silvery Mylar paper, which looks a little bit like aluminum foil, and gold ribbon. I also always tie or tape or glue a little extra present to the top of the package. On the presents for children, it's usually a lollipop or a small toy. For grown-ups, perhaps a flower or a tiny straw figure, or an amusing little object made of hardened, painted dough (like a Santa Claus or elf, or even a hot dog or hamburger!).

For birthdays or "just because" gifts, I sometimes take plain brown wrapping paper, the kind used for wrapping parcels to be mailed, and write over and over on it, in large letters with a felt-tipped pen, "HAPPY BIRTHDAY TO JEFFREY, HAPPY BIRTHDAY TO JEFFREY," or whatever. I sometimes do the same for anniversary gifts. If I've used a green pen, I tie the package with green velvet ribbon; with a red pen, red ribbon, and so on.

If a package is small enough, I might wrap it in a scarf (I secure it with transparent tape) and tie it with yarn.

It's fun to wrap cylindrical-shaped gifts so that they look like a child's birthday "popper" with ribbon and a "grill" at each end.

Another thing that's fun to do when you're sending a very small gift—a pillbox, cuff links, a charm for someone's bracelet—is to put it in a tiny box, put the tiny box in a slightly bigger one, put that one in a slightly bigger one, and so on and on. The final box should be *very* large. (This one may not be worth the effort if you can't be around to watch it being unwrapped.)

What to Buy for the Person Who "Has Everything"

Every year at Christmas, in among the department store ads in the newspapers, you'll always find a few ads, usually placed by the more prestigious stores in town, suggesting gifts "for the person who has everything." And what kind of items are offered? Solid gold paperclips. Platinum toothpicks. Once I saw an ad for an electric tie rack. It's meant to be hung in the closet. When a man wants to select a tie, he pushes a button, a light goes on, and the ties revolve around a kind of conveyor belt, which he can stop when he sees a tie he thinks he might want to wear. The light allows him to examine it more closely.

(In a slightly different category is the diamond clip someone once gave me for my ponytail. It's beautiful, but it tends to come undone and it doesn't hold my hair back as securely as the elastic-covered ponytail holders you can buy in the dime store. So I keep it in the vault along with all the other jewelry I don't wear very often.)

Though no one's ever given me a revolving tie rack, I've had my share of gold paperclips and platinum toothpicks, and I know why people give them to me. They say to themselves (and sometimes they say it directly to me) that it's impossible to buy any other kind of gift for me because I'm one of those people who has everything.

They're only partly right. There are very few material possessions that I *need,* and the things that I do need I can always go out and buy for myself. But it isn't impossible to buy an interesting, useful gift for me, or anyone else who "has everything," without resorting to solid gold paperclips.

If you know people who already "have everything" and you want to buy gifts for them—or feel that for whatever reason you *must* remember them at Christmas or on birthdays—don't panic. Get the gold paperclip or the gimmicky eye-catching new gadget if you know the person and think he or she will enjoy owning such things. But don't overlook the fact that people who have everything also run out of things—just like people who have less. Wine, coffee, and tea get drunk. Candy, cheese, and nuts get eaten. Scratch pads and stationery get written on. Marking pens and pencils get used up. Books are read and get put away on the shelf.

It would be pointless for me to discuss item by item the long gift list that appeared a few pages back, but anything on the list that people use or enjoy and then run out of makes a great gift even for the person who "has everything."

If the person on your list is a collector of things, get him or her something new to add to the collection. I'm talking about stamps or buttons, or paperweights or little fish (which I collect), or records—not diamonds, fur coats, racehorses, and cars. Obviously.

Any handmade craft item is one-of-a-kind. Which means that the person who "has everything" can't possibly already own it. Areas such as SoHo in New York are marvelous places to shop for one-of-a-kind items. Assuming you know something about the taste of the person you're shopping for, you should have little trouble picking up some moderately priced handmade item that will be just the thing to give to the person who already "has everything." (Look for little ceramic bud vases, silk-screened scarves or T-shirts, belts or change purses of hand-tooled leather, miniature hand-crafted picture frames, quilted patchwork pillows. That sort of thing.)

Finally, are you sure the person who "has everything" really does? For years I didn't own a watch—not because I don't like watches, certainly not because I couldn't afford to buy a watch. I'm not quite sure why I didn't own one except that for a long time I never even thought about wearing one. Then a friend noticed my watchlessness and got me one as a gift. Now I wonder how I ever got along without one.

A watch can be very costly and I'm certainly not suggesting that it's an ideal gift for all the people you know who "have everything." Only that maybe some of those people don't have everything after all.

Phyllis and Bob Wagner got me a black silk umbrella with a silver handle. I treasure it. Someone I know didn't own an umbrella, so I got her one. Someone else was forever complaining about her disorganized desk, so I bought her bright red plastic "In" and "Out" boxes, the kind you see in an office.

It may not be easy to figure out what to give the person who "has everything," but with a little thought and imagination it can be done.

A Few Thoughts about Gifts and Children

Most children enjoy giving gifts almost as much as they like getting them. It makes them feel very grown up and pleased with themselves to be on the giving end of a gift. Certainly their generosity ought to be encouraged.

Unfortunately, a lot of parents deprive their children of some very important parts of the gift-giving experience. I know one father whose small boy wanted to get diamond jewelry for his mother's birthday, maybe because he knew that's what his father sometimes did. Children his age don't know what diamonds cost, of course, and he thought he could buy diamonds with his allowance. The father apparently thought it would be cute to take the boy to Cartier's, have him pick out a piece of jewelry, and present it to his mother. So that's what he did. I don't suppose this boy will really grow up thinking that you can buy diamonds for two dollars, but I'm afraid that with a father like that, the child will have to learn the hard way about what they used to call the value of a dollar.

I know of another child, a little girl, who saved her allowance all year and went out to buy Christmas presents with her grandmother. The little girl had about $15 to spend, five people on her list, and she wanted to buy each of them a pair of gloves. The grandmother headed for the glove department at Saks, where it turned out the little girl discovered that her $15 wasn't quite enough. But the grandmother, instead of explaining to the child why she couldn't get gloves for everybody, helping her to decide on other gifts, and then taking her around to find them, laid out the extra money herself. The other way would have been harder for the grandmother but better for the child.

There isn't anything really wrong with what either of these grownups did, but how much better it would have been if the children had been given the opportunity to practice dealing with money and making choices. I don't think children are ever too young to start learning about such things.

I'll tell you what I used to get from Steven, Jeffrey, and Susan: pictures that they'd drawn themselves; little funny-looking clay ashtrays; pot holders. Things from the dime store bought with money saved from their allowances. I get the same things now from my nieces (plus an occasional bar of strawberry soap or a scented candle). And I love them.

Now that the children are grown, I get very different kinds of presents from them: a computer clock one Mother's Day, a Polaroid camera for Christmas. Their presents to me are usually joint endeavors. They get together and decide on one gift, then each chips in a third of the money. I'm most thrilled with their choice of gifts and pleased with the way they've learned to handle their money.

Getting Your Message Across: Phone Calls, Notes, and Letters

I almost always prefer to pick up the phone rather than write what I have to say. Phoning is easier, quicker, more direct. It's more in line with my personal style.

But there are times when a phone call just won't do, or won't do nearly as well as a handwritten note or letter. The only acceptable way to send condolences, for example, is with a card or note. Notes are also better for saying thank you (for the gift, for the party, for the lovely weekend, or for the kind, considerate thing someone has done for you) because they require more thought and effort than a phone call. They somehow mean more.

Condolences are a difficult kind of note to write because people are so uncomfortable—embarrassed, almost—at the idea of death. It's easier to buy a card with a printed message. A handwritten note is more personal, though, and always a better way to express your sympathy. You needn't worry about brilliance of style. A few simple, sincere words—that your thoughts are with the family, that you're greatly saddened by their loss—are quite enough.

Thank-you notes are easier, at least they're easier for me because they can be more spontaneous. I usually dash them off from the top of my head—the first thing that comes to mind is what goes down on the paper. I think the trick with thank-you notes is to write them immediately when the gift or the experience is still fresh in your mind.

Another reason for writing immediately, of course, is to get the job over and done with. I know for myself that if I put off writing a thank-you note even for a few days, I may forget about it altogether. Thank-you notes are much too important to be forgotten. As much fun as it is to receive gifts, I've always felt that they are a responsibility. When I accept a present, I'm also accepting the responsibility of writing to thank the person who sent it. (It's a concept I feel very strongly about and I've done my best to pass it on to my children.)

The message—what you say in a note or letter—is the important part. But don't forget that your choice of stationery or notepaper says something about you too. I have a whole "wardrobe" of stationery and notepaper in different styles and colors and I like to write with colored pens—a green pen with white and green paper, a dark brown pen with beige or off-white paper. But the stationery I use most often is a medium Wedgwood blue, with my signature, "Lyn," embossed in white across one corner. I didn't know stationery could have sex appeal, but apparently this kind does. Not one but *two* men commented on "that sexy stationery." (I think what they really meant is that it's very pretty.)

There are so many different styles, colors, textures, and even shapes to choose from now, you should have no trouble finding stationery that is expressive of your own personal style—simple and elegant if that's what you want; eye-catching and dramatic; charmingly feminine. Choose the kind that best gets your message across.

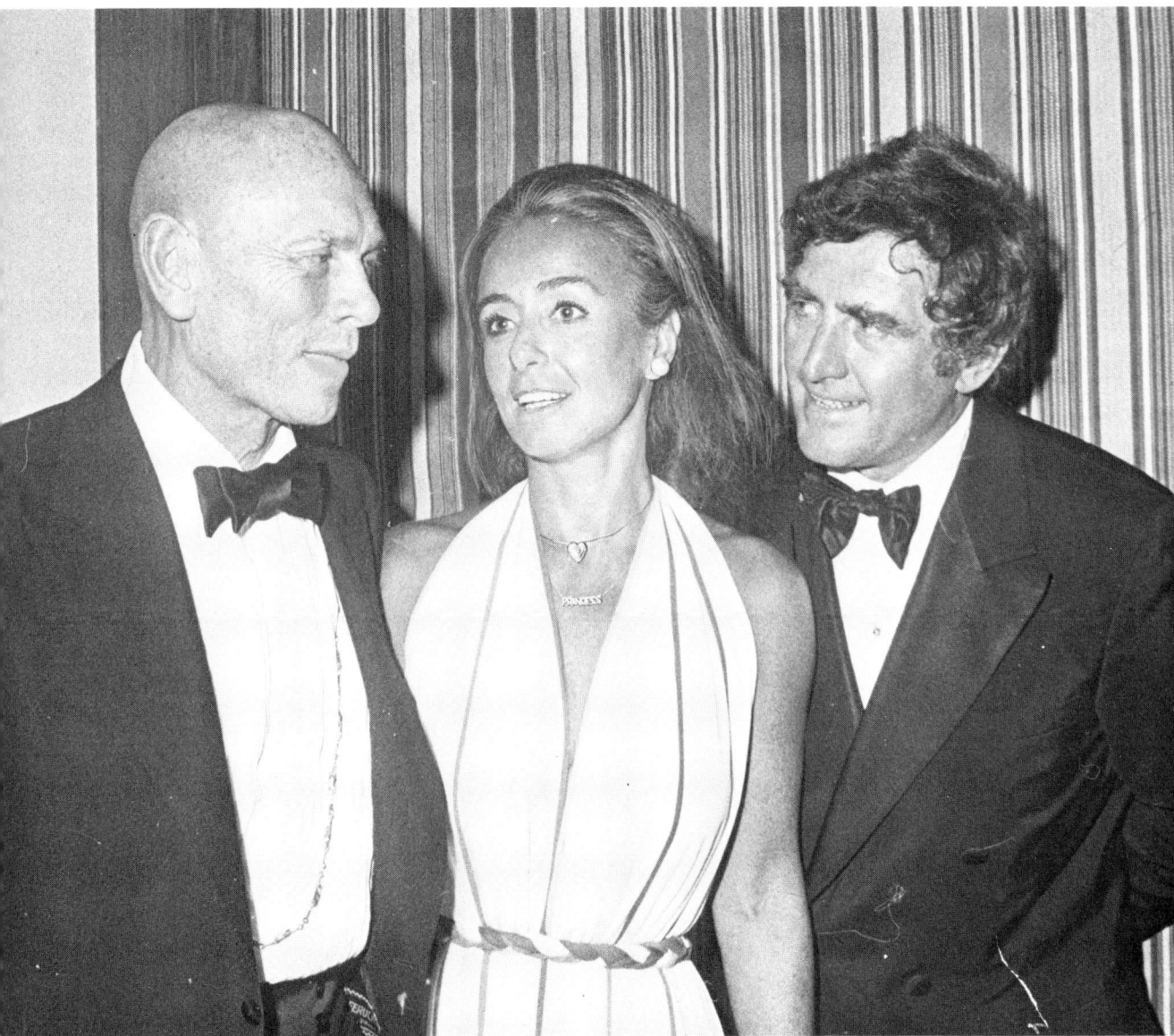

Yul Brynner, star, and Lee Guber, producer, of *The King and I*. Here we all are, at the opening in May 1977. (PHOTO: METROPOLITAN PHOTO SERVICE, INC.)

5

Managing

Living with style doesn't just "happen." A life with style may appear to be easy, spontaneous, even glamorous. That's the way it's supposed to look. But in truth it requires paying attention to detail. Planning, organizing, and following through. "Managing," in other words. Managing time, money, and energy.

We often hear people describe others as "having a mind for detail," or "a talent for organization," or "a knack for getting things done," as though these abilities are something you're either born with or not. Not so! I think "managing" is one of those learnable skills, like swimming or needlepoint. If you really want to, you can.

You can master the big and little details of your life—like party planning, packing for trips, overseeing helpers, making sure that whatever needs doing gets done and gets done well. And you can do it without being swamped in the process.

First Things First

With what I've just said about paying attention to detail, it may seem contradictory for me to suggest "putting first things first." The truth is, it's hardly possible to give *anything* the time and effort it deserves until you've decided where it belongs on your list of priorities. Wouldn't it be foolish to lavish attention on the overly fussy and trivial while the important is left undone? And isn't it just as unproductive to continue to wrestle doggedly with problems or situations that are beyond your control while ignoring the things that you *can* change for the better?

I've never had a complex that makes me feel I need to do twenty different things at once and do them all well. I know I have to focus on the one thing that's most important at the moment, whatever it might be; once I've grappled with that, everything else miraculously falls into place.

This is all very abstract. Perhaps I'd better put my "first things first" way into more concrete terms. Let's say I wake up one rainy morning only to discover that the roof is leaking. I also notice that the tulips delivered by the florist the day before are badly wilted. Flowers have more style than roofs; they're prettier and I like them better. But a leaky roof, when you have to live with it, is more important than wilted flowers. So my first priority is to have the leak taken care of. I call the building management to let them know that my roof needs fixing. Only then do I ring up the florist to find out how to revive wilting tulips. (Incidentally, the florist says to plunge the stems of drooping tulips into a bowl of ice cubes and cold water; within a couple of hours, the tulips stand erect and proud.)

More to the point with regard to the following pages is the "first things first" way to plan a party. Place cards, imaginative centerpieces, and the glow of polished silver are important. Special touches like these are part of living with style. But in the end it seems that no amount of attention paid to special touches makes up for poor planning in the guest department. People make the party. So my top party-planning priority is the guest list.

How to Plan a No-Fail (or Almost) Party Guest List

Obviously, you don't have to think much about a guest list if you're simply inviting one other couple over for dinner (or for drinks before the theater or supper afterward). But if you're planning any gathering of, say, six or more, it's a good idea to give some thought to the people mix. It's almost like chemistry. You can't always predict the results, but they're more likely to be good if you think about each person or couple in terms of what they'll add to the evening.

For example, it's always nice to have one or two "entertainers" on hand. No, I don't mean professional clowns or show people or even life-of-the-party types. I do mean men and women who are gregarious and have an amusing way with an anecdote.

It's also a good idea to try to have people whose interests and occupations are varied. I think it's a mistake to plan a party where everyone is in the same line of work. Endless shoptalk may be the result. At a party consisting of twenty conservative Republicans, or eight happily married suburban couples between the ages of thirty-five and forty, the potential for lively interaction is somewhat limited.

I'd also avoid inviting two superstars to the same party—two tennis pros, for example, or two trial lawyers, or two novelists, or two top executives from competing companies. If it somehow worked out that way, I'd try to seat them at different tables.

Obviously, it's better not to invite people who you know don't get along or whose relationship with one another is potentially explosive. (I say "obviously," but some hostesses seem to relish the idea of such high-voltage combinations as a man, his wife, and his mistress; a woman, her husband, and her lover; an actor and the critic who said he couldn't act his way out of a paper bag; or any two people who, for whatever reason, might be expected to clash.)

A good mix also depends on what kind of evening you're planning and why. Do you simply want to spend relaxed social time with friends? Is the party really a means of reciprocating—entertaining in return for being entertained? Is it to be a "special event" party (a birthday party, for example, or a party to introduce new people to your neighborhood or club)? Or perhaps the party is just for you to enjoy entertaining (or because you feel you *should* entertain every once in a while). In any event, your reason for planning the party will determine, at least in part, whom to invite.

People who see each other constantly often don't add up to a lively gathering. Though it can be very pleasant to spend an evening with close friends, it's amazing how the little dinner for six or eight changes in character when at least one of the couples is new to the others. New faces alter the chemistry of the group, add an element of freshness and even suspense; nobody knows what they're going to say or do and everyone is anxious to find out.

If your reason for planning a party is mainly a matter of reciprocating, then obviously you're going to invite many of the people who have entertained you in the past. If possible, though, I'd avoid ending up with a roomful of total strangers. Making sure that everyone has been properly introduced to everyone else is hard enough. Harder still is getting in that little "tag line" that provides your guests with the conversational lead they need to get started talking with one another. (You know: "Mr. and Mrs. Smith, this is Mr. and Mrs. Jones. Mr. and Mrs. Jones are just in from Houston.") Better to have at least a few people who know each other well enough to need no introductions or conversational tag lines.

For a birthday or anniversary party, you will, of course, invite people who are close to the guest(s) of honor, including perhaps members of the family. Obvious? Yes, indeed. Except that I remember one evening, ostensibly a birthday party for a woman I know. The hostess apparently got sidetracked halfway through the guest list because a good 50 percent of the people at the party were strangers to the guest of honor (but well known to the hostess herself).

There's no way to guarantee good chemistry at a party, but you can increase the probability of everyone's having a marvelous time if you don't leave your guest list to chance.

Party Food: Serving with Style

There are excellent books to help you plan the food for your parties, large or small, simple or elaborate. I'm not talking about cookbooks per se, but books suggesting recipes *and* menus for an entire festive meal from beginning to end. If you're a novice at menu planning, these books can be invaluable. Even if you're an experienced hostess they can be a big help, since almost everyone draws an occasional blank when the question of what to serve comes up. One of my favorite books is *Great Dinners from* Life; published in 1969, it's what's sometimes referred to as an "oldie but goodie." Another marvelous book of recipes and menus is the *New York Times Menu Cook Book* by Craig Claiborne.

A good general rule about party food is: the larger the group, the fewer and simpler should be the items on the menu. I think this applies even when you have helpers to do the cooking and serving for you. It makes particular sense when you and you alone are in charge of the whole show.

If you're totally without help, or if it's a huge party and you have only one or two people to help you, then you certainly should consider food that lends itself to being served buffet-style (always quicker and less complicated than having to rely on waiters—or you—to go around serving every guest).

If a buffet is your choice, try to plan a menu around food that can be served cold or at room temperature or can be kept hot for a while in covered dishes without losing flavor. Avoid anything that needs tricky, last-minute preparation. (This usually includes any recipe that ends with the breathless injunction to "serve immediately.")

Buffet-style service isn't necessarily any less elegant or "correct" than having waiters serve your guests at their places—though it is obviously less formal.

What about a caterer? A good caterer can take much of the pressure off you, obviously, and sometimes it's the only way to go. Do make an attempt to find the very *best* caterer available. (One way is to ask around among your friends.)

At a recent party for eighty, which I planned in honor of my friend Lee Guber's birthday, there was a main course of veal, fettucine, and sautéed zucchini. It was preceded by shrimp in mustard sauce, and followed up by coffee, cheese, fruit, and birthday cake.

(The cake, incidentally, was ordered from a place called Creative Cakes on East 74th Street in New York. If you bring them a picture, they'll do a "portrait" in cake, "painting" it in with icing of different colors. The only picture I had of Lee showed him in a tuxedo with black bow tie. The likeness that came back was startling. There he was—Lee served up on an enormous cake plate, tuxedo, bow tie, and all.

(Serving a portrait cake isn't the kind of thing to do too often. I've only done it once, and I would imagine that by the second or third time around, the idea loses much of its "punch.")

There are food fads just as there are fads in practically everything else. For a while, it seems everyone is serving bouillabaisse. Other times it's crown roast of lamb. I enjoy any good-tasting food, but when I have a party I always try to serve something just a little bit unexpected and out of the ordinary.

One of my favorite recent menus was planned around a piquant choucroute garni—which is really sauerkraut, smoked pork butt, Polish kielbasa, knockwurst, bratwurst, and veal sausages elevated to the nth degree. With it, we had stuffed eggplant, paella, and a salad. For dessert, there was lemon mousse with strawberries, and a bowl of fresh fruit. (I think it's always a good idea to include fruit as part of the dessert; many people appreciate something light after a hearty, rich meal.)

At a recent pretheater get-together for six people, including *New York Times* columnist John Corry and Jean Vanderbilt, actor John Gavin and his wife Constance Towers, Lee Guber and myself, the menu included shrimp in mustard sauce, an assortment of cheeses, wine and beer—just enough to tide us over until supper at ten thirty or so. Everything was set out on a table. People served themselves.

I dislike fussy little hors d'oeuvres consisting of bits and pieces and dribs and drabs of different things spread on crackers. I'm more likely to serve crudités—fresh raw vegetables such as cauliflower, broccoli, cherry tomatoes, etc., cut into bite-size pieces and served cold with a variety of sauces to dip them in.

Possibly my very favorite first course of all is shrimp with mustard sauce. It has a marvelous taste with just a hint of a "bite" to it, it's easy to make, and I want to pass the recipe on to you.

You'll need:

2 1/2 pounds shrimp, shelled and deveined
1/4 cup finely chopped parsley
1/4 cup finely chopped shallots
1/4 cup tarragon vinegar
1/4 cup wine vinegar
1/2 cup olive oil
4 tablespoons Dijon mustard
2 teaspoons crushed red peppers
2 teaspoons salt
Freshly ground black pepper

Mix together in a large bowl—everything but the shrimp. Then pour over the shrimp and toss gently. And that's it. The recipe is enough for twelve people when served on plates as a first course. Or it could be passed around as an hors d'oeuvre, to be speared on toothpicks.

One of my favorite ways of entertaining a few close friends is the "cooking" party: each person—or couple—brings the ingredients of part of the meal, and we all cook together in my kitchen. At a recent "cooking party," Phyllis Wagner baked bread and made a fabulous pasta dish that is a specialty of hers. Lee Guber, who is a real gourmet cook, did "Veal Neapolitan," veal with proscuitto and mozzarella cheese with a tomato base. I made—what else?—shrimp in mustard sauce. Susan Fine made a cake. (Bob Wagner and Bill Fine—who didn't cook—were off in another room talking about who knows what while the four of us were busy in the kitchen. Maybe it's a good thing they were. Though it's a good size, my kitchen wouldn't have accommodated six chefs at once. As it is, I need at least two more stoves.)

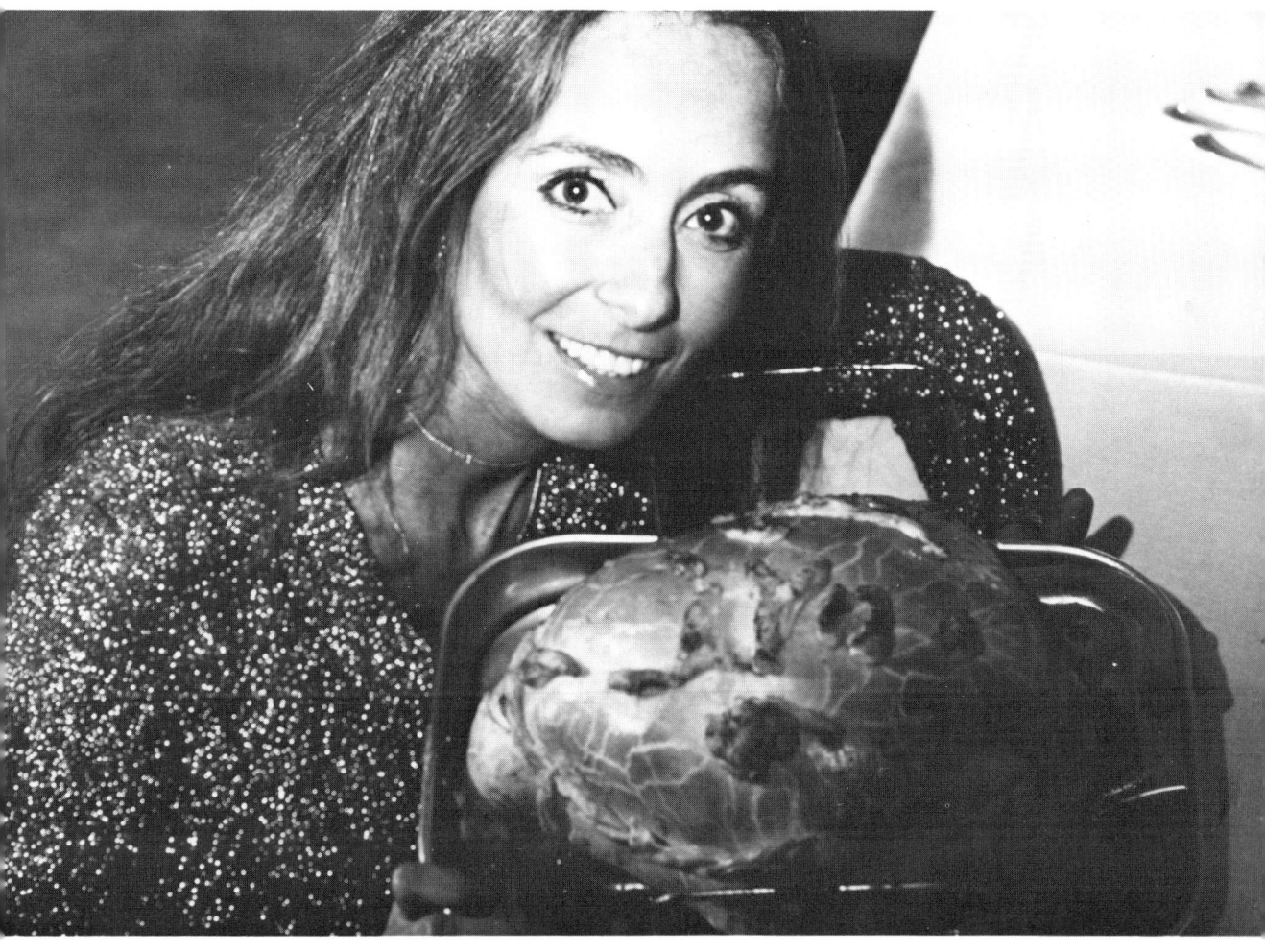

The ham *en croûte* with my name on it (look closely), made for me by a friend. (PHOTO: LEE GUBER)

Another good party idea is to have each person or couple bring a finished dish. A lot of people I know have been entertaining this way lately and it's marvelous because it means less work for the hostess. At the same time it allows guests to show off their culinary expertise. (As hostess, however, you *do* need to coordinate things so that you don't end up with a meal consisting of four salads and five desserts.)

A couple of years ago I went to a somewhat different kind of cooking party—or maybe I should call it a cooking *contest*. Restaurant consultant George Lang was the host. The food of the hour was chili. Everyone made chili at home and brought it to the party. Each chili got a number and all the guests sampled and rated them one by one. Then a vote was taken and a winner named. I cooked with a friend.

Our chili was sensational, even if I do say so myself. About forty different steps were required and we had to start cooking early the day before. Even so, it wasn't good enough. We came in eighth. The chili made by famous chef Jim Beard didn't do that well either. He placed fifth. The winner and chili-making champion of the evening was, in fact, George Lang, the host.

Organizing for a Party—Step by Step by Step

What do you do after you've decided whom to invite and what to serve? Make lists.

First a master shopping list which includes all the ingredients for all the food on the menu that you or your help will be cooking for the party. Don't forget to include wine, liquor, club soda, and anything else you'll need for cocktails before dinner, as well as Cognac, brandy, or liqueurs for after dinner. (If you're using a caterer, find out from him or her what you should supply yourself and put *those* items on a list.)

Next, divide the master food list into other lists. Everything you need from the supermarket goes on one list. Wine and liquor go on another. If you use a butcher, as I do, you'll need a third list for meats. Cheeses and other items that you buy from a specialty food store go on a fourth list. Fresh fruits and vegetables, if you buy them at a greengrocer, go on a fifth list. And so on.

(The point of listing foods separately, according to where you're going to buy them, is, of course, so that you can go into each market or shop and know at a glance what you need. As you buy each item, check it off the list.)

Once again, read carefully through all the recipes to make sure you have all the necessary pots, pans, utensils, and other equipment. List what you need to buy.

Check through your china and linen closets to see if you have an adequate supply of dishes (including bowls and platters for serving), wine glasses, napkins, tablecloths, etc. Whatever is missing goes on still another list. This is also the time to make a note to yourself, or your housekeeper if you have one, that the silver needs polishing, or that folded linen needs pressing, etc.

Now think about table and seating arrangements. If you're planning a very large party, you may need to rent extra tables and chairs. Most cities have party rental services where for a moderate price you can get all the tables and chairs (and coat racks, dishes, linen, glassware, and chafing dishes) you may need.

(When I was planning the party for eighty mentioned earlier, I had to rent eighty chairs and ten round tables. But then I was immediately confronted by another problem: how to fit all those tables and chairs into my apartment. My decorator, Mark Hampton, came up with the idea of hiring movers to come and clear away the furniture from my living room and dining room and load it into a van. This was done the day of the party. With the furniture removed, there was plenty of space for the tables and chairs. Next morning, my furniture, which had spent the night in the van at a warehouse, was replaced.)

This is also the time to decide whether you want or need outside helpers. Depending on the size of the party and how much you want to invest, you may want to consider hiring a waiter to pass hors d'oeuvres and to serve at the buffet table. A bartender. Someone to help you—or to take over completely—in the kitchen. Someone to answer the door and take coats.

You may be able to get along just fine without any of these helpers, but it's wise to keep in mind that they are available if you need them. To locate help for a party call a domestic employment agency.

What about music? I occasionally hire musicians, but some people don't feel their parties are complete without a pianist or a guitar player or one or two other people to provide music for dancing.

If you do want live music, arrange for it as quickly as possible. Many musicians are booked months in advance. Your best bet for locating musicians is to ask around among your friends for the names of people who've played at their parties. Another idea is to phone your local musicians' union. Or look in the Yellow Pages under "Musicians."

About now you should also be giving some thought to centerpieces, place cards, flowers, and other special touches. I rather like the idea of edible centerpieces, and for that party of eighty which I keep referring back to, I asked florist Robert Webb, an ingenious young man, to see what he could come up with. The results were sensational: for each table he made a kind of "container" out of the most perfect, fresh, unblemished asparagus he could find; the stalks were tied together in a circular shape. Inside each "container" he piled artichokes, cauliflower, eggplant, and other vegetables. He also used hollowed-out artichokes as candle holders. It all looked quite lovely on the pale green tablecloths, and nothing went to waste. Guests took the vegetables home.

A basket heaped with big yellow lemons makes an attractive centerpiece. So do three or four potted geraniums or African violets or other flowering plants grouped at the center of a table. At the party where choucroute garni was served, I filled enormous earthenware bowls with sauerkraut and piled pickles and brilliant red and green tomatoes on top.

One thing always to keep in mind about centerpieces: they shouldn't obstruct your guests' view of one another. Centerpieces that are short and fat (or tall and thin) are best.

I've always enjoyed devising pretty or amusing place cards. For one dinner party I bought miniature potted orchid plants and set one at every place. Each plant had a small tag attached; on the back was the Latin name for the plant; on the front I wrote the name of the guest. For my son Steven's twenty-fifth birthday party, which was large but mostly family, I managed to find a small photograph of each guest. Then I went out and bought picture frames from the five-and-ten. Each photograph was framed and became a place card.

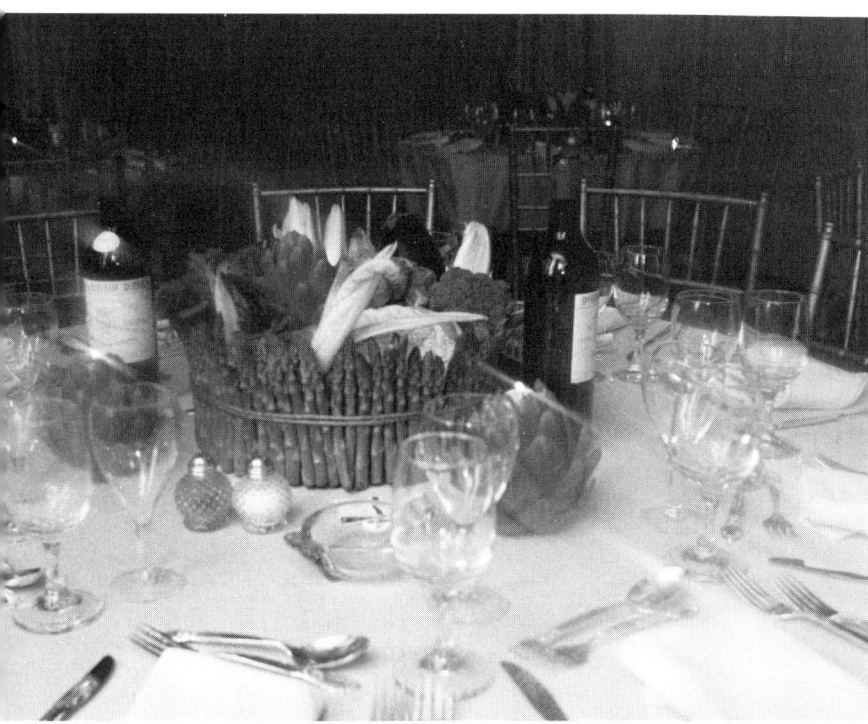

The vegetable centerpiece and the artichoke candle holders at a large dinner party. (PHOTO: SAL TRIANA)

Kitty Carlisle Hart looks at the cake portrait of Lee Guber at the same dinner party. (PHOTO: SAL TRIANA)

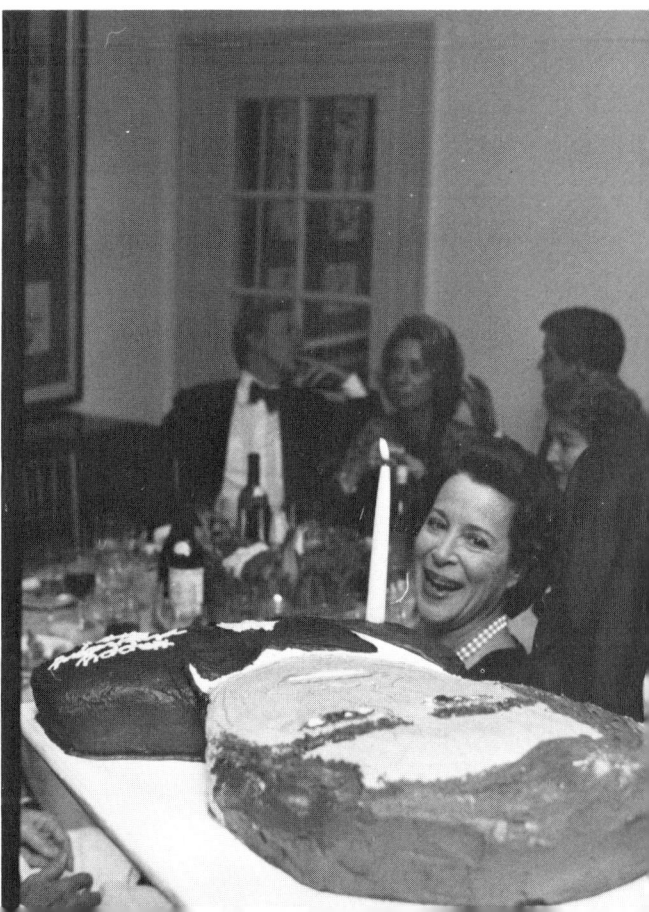

SHOPPING: The sooner you can buy, rent, or arrange for most of the things on your various lists, the better. (Perishable items, of course, are the exception; these should be bought no sooner than the day before the party.)

Never underestimate the convenience of telephone ordering. I can't think of any good reason why you personally should have to select Coke and club soda, paper towels, milk, butter, eggs, flour, or canned or frozen grocery items (unless, of course, the stores in your area don't deliver). Phoning is quicker and just as good if you tell the person on the other end of the line the exact size and quantity of everything you need and specify brand-name products, if they're important to you.

Of course, it sometimes happens that the person you speak to doesn't take your order down correctly—or passes it on to someone else to fill. As a result, there may be a mistake or two in the delivery. That's when your list really comes in handy. Each time a phone order is delivered to my house either my housekeeper Elizabeth or I check to make sure that each item ordered has been delivered. If something is missing, or if I've ordered, say, College Inn chicken broth and some other kind has been delivered, one of us calls to say so and to ask them to send the delivery person back with the missing (or correct) items.

Some items—fruits, vegetables, meats, cheeses, etc.—should be hand-picked. I always shop for these myself because I want to see what I'm getting—and also because I enjoy it. For fruits and vegetables I go to Perrone's on Third Avenue and 65th Street. They have the biggest, most beautiful specimens of every fruit and vegetable imaginable, including out-of-season produce that's hard to find anywhere else.

Before I shop for meat, I check in Jacques Pépin's book *La Technique* so that I'll know what to look for in the particular cut I'm buying.

COOKING: The more you can do ahead of time, the fresher and less hassled you'll feel when it's time to serve—and the more you'll enjoy your own party. Some dishes, as you probably know, actually improve if they're cooked ahead and allowed to sit a day or so in the refrigerator before serving. Things like crepes can be made and frozen several days in advance. Other food really must be cooked just prior to serving, but even then you may be able to simplify your life during those crucial hours just before dinner when so many things need to be done at once by doing as much as you can of the chopping, peeling, measuring out, and assembling of ingredients in advance. Tie your hair back, roll up your sleeves, and if there are people around to help you out, hand out the aprons and ask them to do just that.

Countdown for Thanksgiving dinner. I always tie my hair back and dress comfortably when I cook. (PHOTO: LEE GUBER)

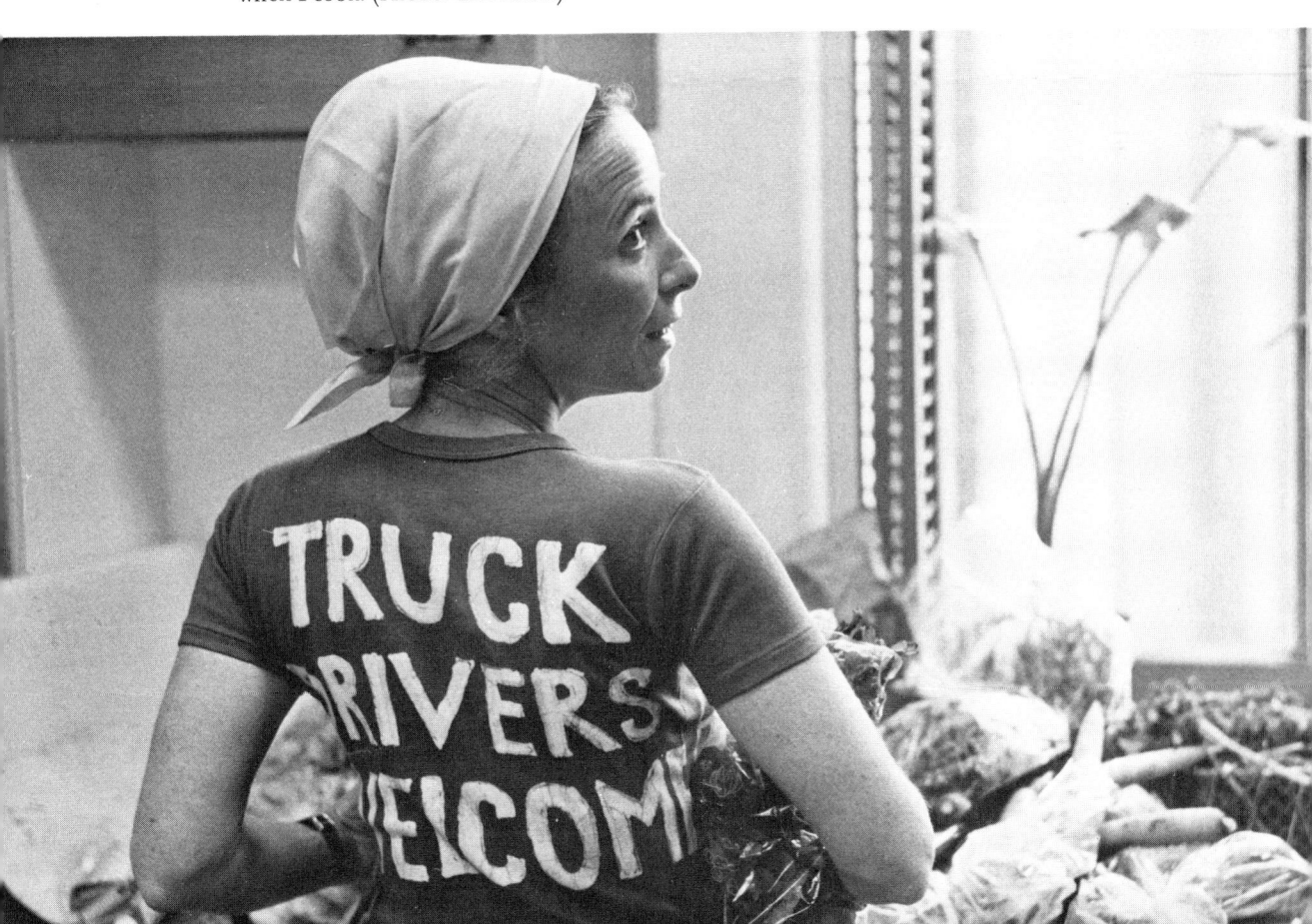

Children at the Table?

Children, of course, will be present on family occasions and religious holidays. In fact, we plan many of these events especially *for* the children. At such times, it's fun and enjoyable for adults and children alike when everyone is seated at the same table. The children, like little monkeys, ape the adults' table manners and learn to contribute to the conversation—often in the most outrageous, hilarious ways. Their comments sometimes "make" the party.

I think you'll agree that children are out of place at most grown-up parties. They get bored with adult talk, and their fussing and fidgeting is annoying to everyone seated near them. When you're having a grown-up party, try to arrange to have your children tucked away in bed shortly after the guests arrive.

If for some reason that isn't possible, set up a small table in a corner of the room for the kids. Everyone will be happier.

The Helpers in Your Life and How to Work with Them

The best way to find a good housekeeper or cook or maid or chauffeur—or help of any kind—is to call the top domestic employment agency in your area and tell them exactly what kind of person (or persons) you have in mind. Good agencies have a reputation to maintain. It's to their advantage to screen thoroughly and to rate as well as they can the abilities of all the people who come to them for employment. (You could also place an ad in the newspaper. But then you'd have to do the screening and rating yourself.)

The agency will send prospective employees to your home for you to interview. By all means ask the person (let's assume it's a woman) why she left her last job. If her explanation isn't clear or doesn't make sense, tell her you don't understand and ask her to go over it again. Also, make sure to ask for references and phone or write to check on them before you make a final decision.

One of the main reasons for such an interview is so that you can explain the job in detail. If you expect the person you hire to mind the children, clean, cook, do all the washing and ironing, answer the telephone and the door, take care of pets and plants, and do all the marketing as well, let her know. That way, she will have the opportunity to accept or decline these responsibilities and there will be fewer misunderstandings later on.

It's up to you to stick to your end of the bargain, too, and not ask her—once she's safely hired and dependent on you for her livelihood—to also hang wallpaper, move heavy furniture, or run the elevator in your building when the regular operators are on strike.

If her references are in order, if she understands what's required of her and is willing and able to do the work, and if you *like* her (this last is very important, at least to me; I want to feel good about the people who work for me—it's very unpleasant to have to deal day in and day out with someone you dislike), then hire her.

Your relationships with the people who work for you are personal. You have to find your own way of dealing with each other and the jobs to be done. But if the situation as it is leaves something to be desired, there are a couple of things you can do to help improve it.

Make lists. I want to say that Elizabeth and the other people who work for me are wonderful. They always have been. But there are times when we all benefit from lists. At those times I use a little pad and write in it everything that has to be done, (1), (2), (3), in the order it has to be done. You can't expect anyone to be able to read your mind—not even your husband or best friend, let alone someone who's just come to work for you. When you put things down on paper in their order of priority, no one needs to read your mind.

Incidentally, I think it's important that children not get into the habit of thinking that anything they don't want to do, the housekeeper or maid can or should do for them. For one thing, the children may not always have a housekeeper or maid (at this point in their lives, *my* children certainly don't). More important, it robs them of the opportunity to learn responsibility.

There was no maid when Steven, Jeffrey, and Susan were little, but I did have a nurse for them. When the boys were six and seven (they're sixteen months apart) and Susan three, I decided it was time they started to take care of their toys, putting them up on the shelves when they were finished playing. I told them what I expected them to do.

"But the nurse can do it," they insisted. And I would insist, "No, the nurse is not here to pick up toys. She feeds you and looks after you when I'm away. It's your job to pick up the toys because the toys belong to you." And it would start all over again: "But the nurse can do it. . . ."

I finally handled it by telling them that every day just before dinner I would come to their room and say, "Toys up on the shelves in fifteen minutes" (and I'd show them the clock). Then in fifteen minutes, any toys not put away would go out the back door.

And that's the way it was three days in a row. Wednesday, Thursday, Friday, toys out the back door. Gone. On the fourth day, the toy supply had dwindled considerably and I think they finally got the idea that indeed the nurse was not responsible for their things, because when I went in and said, "Toys up in fifteen minutes," they went running and scuttling like three little beavers.

Yes, I certainly do know that not everyone has a maid or housekeeper or nurse for their children. But every one of us has to deal with other kinds of "helpers"—cabdrivers, cleaners, painters, carpenters; people who repair appliances, hang wallpaper, install flooring, deliver packages. The list could go on and on. And then there are the people who own and work in the shops where we buy things. How well we manage often depends on how promptly, efficiently, and well they do their jobs.

Some jobs are easier or more glamorous or more financially rewarding than others. My feeling is that *all* jobs are important, and so are the men and women who do them. The people who aren't good at their jobs have my sympathy. I assume they're unhappy about their work. They may be locked into jobs they don't really want to do. Their helplessness makes them miserable, angry. I understand.

Even so, I don't want to be a victim of surliness and incompetence.

I'd rather deal—who wouldn't?—with people who do their jobs well and deliver on time.

That's why I've always made an effort to seek out and stay with the people who do the best work. It's not always easy to find these people. (In fact, too much of my time is spent phoning around to friends and acquaintances asking whether they know of a good cleaner or an air-conditioner repairman who can be counted on to get the job done before the cold weather sets in.)

When I do find someone who does good work and does it quickly, his name (or the company name) and phone number gets filed in a little box in my kitchen.

I tell the person how much I appreciate the work. (Sometimes I wonder if they know how much I *really* mean it.) If they're working long hours inside the house, I make sure Elizabeth, my maid, offers them coffee or, if it's hot, something cold to drink. I become a loyal and devoted fan. I don't hesitate to share my good fortune. I often pass these names along to friends and tell my friends to make sure to say, "Mrs. Revson says you're the best in the business." (It's a way of making things a little bit better for everyone: my friends, the "helpers" in question, and me.)

The point is that it's well worth your while to get to know, and cultivate relationships with, the people who do the best work. They deserve your business. The incompetents don't. And maybe in time the incompetents will get the message—right in the pocketbook, where it counts.

Nobody's perfect, right? Everyone makes an occasional mistake, even the best, most competent people. I think it's a good idea to allow for occasional slip-ups, but only up to a point. I try to adhere to a one-two-three-strikes-you're-out policy. In other words, a couple of mistakes are unfortunate, but tolerable. (When someone has disappointed me, I do always make a point of saying—as nicely as possible —that I understand but I hope it won't happen again.) Three are too many, though. Especially when it comes to being ripped off.

I always go over my grocery bills to make sure they've been added up correctly, that no charge has been made for undelivered items, and that the prices are in line with what I know is reasonable. Unfortunately, in certain neighborhoods—mine is one of them—"accidental overcharging" is far from rare. I remember once being billed $60 (yes!) for six apples (the store said they meant it to be 60 cents). Another time I ordered and was charged for four pounds of shrimp, but the package felt light and sure enough, the shrimp weighed out at two pounds on my kitchen scale.

I suppose the assumption is that people with a certain amount of money don't bother to check their bills because the money is unimportant to them. That's wrong. No one wants to be taken advantage of.

At the same time, some people with a "certain amount of money" are afraid of being thought "petty" if they make a point of checking their bills and calling any mistakes to the attention of the manager of the store or company that sent the bill. I think that's wrong, too. Or maybe "foolish" is a better word.

The way to deal with the helpers in your life is with consideration and respect. We all deserve the same kind of consideration and respect in return.

Quick Getaways: How to Pack like a Pro

Sometimes, if you're going to get away at all, you have to get away quickly: pack on the spur of the moment, jump on a plane, and be off.

I've got the packing part of it down to a system. It involves (among other things) always keeping several clear zippered plastic envelopes full of essentials ready to go in a Hermès canvas bag.

In one clear plastic bag go full-size bottles, tubes, jars, etc., of all the makeup I use at home. I have two of everything; one set on my dressing table, the other packed away in a valise.

A second bag holds hair stuff: brush, combs to comb with and a variety of decorative combs to hold my hair back, barrettes, ponytail holders, bobby pins, etc.

Bag number three is for what I suppose are called "toiletries":

Lubriderm Lotion, No More Tears shampoo, deodorant, Eyenet eye makeup remover, Ultima II After Sun Moisture Balm, Sea & Ski Lipsaver (for sunburn protection, I put it on my lips *and* my nose), etc.

The fourth plastic bag is for emergencies. In it go Band-Aids, aspirin, an antiseptic lotion for cuts and bruises, Tampax, etc.

Bag number five is a smaller one for toothpaste and a toothbrush.

These clear plastic zippered envelopes that you can get at any five-and-ten aren't the greatest in terms of chic but they have one important advantage over the very beautiful Porthault terry cloth: I can see at a glance the contents of each bag without opening it up and peering and pawing through the stuff inside.

Also in my permanently packed valise are a magnifying mirror in a zippered case; a hair dryer; a curling iron (which I've never quite learned how to operate, but I keep trying); a manicure set; a bottle of Woolite. And a marvelous contraption that I got from Hammacher Schlemmer (the best gadget store in New York). This contraption is about the size of a large flashlight and like some big flashlights even has a handle on it. You unscrew the top, fill it up with water to a special mark in the base, plug it in, and within minutes steam comes gushing out—steam that you can use to freshen and unwrinkle your clothes after they're unpacked and hung up on hangers. This gadget is a great improvement over the old turn-on-the-shower-and-steam-your-clothes-in-the-bathroom method. Any woman who travels without a personal maid and an ironing board should have one of them.

As I've mentioned, all of the above are permanently packed in a valise. This saves me the time and trouble (not to mention the brain-racking of trying not to forget anything important) of having to run around collecting and packing travel essentials on the eve of a trip.

(When I come back home again, one of the first things Elizabeth does is to check through all the plastic envelopes to see if anything is used up or missing—I usually leave something behind. These she replaces immediately so that all systems are go for the next time I leave town.)

What about clothes?

A basic travel wardrobe for, say, four days at a warm-weather resort (or at someone's summer house) would include the following:

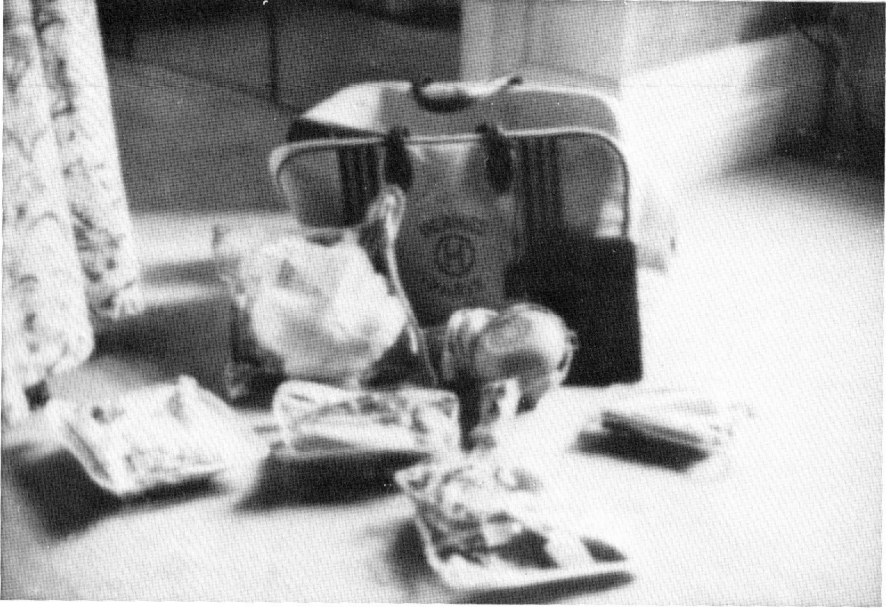

I've simplified my packing by keeping cosmetics, toiletries, and other travel necessities always ready to go in plastic see-through bags. (PHOTO: JEFFREY SHERESKY)

2 pairs of white cotton duck or linen pants. You *could* get by with only one pair, but then what if a zipper breaks or a seam rips?

(Or a pair of white pants and a jumpsuit.)

1 pair of jeans.

3 or 4 T-shirts. (One of them should be special enough so that when teamed with the white pants, they make an outfit that you can wear to restaurants or parties. I often pack a rhinestone-studded sweater by Adolfo.)

1 cotton T-shirt dress, long or short. (Long would take you out at night to dinner or a party; short would be better for sightseeing or lunches in nearby towns, or to wear on the plane to and from your destination. Take your pick, or if you have room, take one of each.)

1 pair of sandals.

1 pair of sneakers.

2 bathing suits.

2 tennis dresses or 2 pairs of white shorts and white tops. (But only if tennis will be on the agenda.)

A terry cloth robe and something to sleep in.

Underwear.

If you pack Woolite, as I do, you can rinse out lingerie and socks as necessary and get into fresh things every day.

I also always pack a plastic bag. (In it go my wet bathing suit or tennis dress—which is always soaked with perspiration by the time I'm finished playing—if there's no time to dry them before catching a flight home.)

Finally, a raincoat or slicker. I hate to pack one but whenever I don't, it rains and I end up having to buy one.

A basic cold-weather wardrobe, for when you're flying off to spend four or five days in another town, would include the following:

1 pair of slacks and a sweater to travel in. Top them off with a fur coat or good cloth coat.

1 skirt in a color that works with the sweater.

1 knit dress—either silk knit or sheer wool jersey. Either is wonderfully "packable," folds small, and doesn't wrinkle easily.

1 silk blouse to wear with the skirt or slacks.

1 long matte jersey dress for parties and dressed-up dinners. PLUS, if you have one, a flat-knit suit that can be worn with the silk blouse for a pulled-together daytime look, and without the blouse for restaurants, theater evenings, etc.

Chains, scarves, belts to accessorize all of the above (except for the long dress).

A comfortable pair of daytime shoes. (Wear them on the plane.)

A pair of high-heeled shoes in tan or beige to wear on more dressed-up occasions.

A terry cloth robe and something to sleep in.

Underwear.

A raincoat.

Either wardrobe will just about fit into a standard twenty-six-inch canvas valise (though I must admit, there are times when I have to sit on the valise and have somebody else zip it closed). Any leftovers can go into a smaller duffle bag.

A few packing tips: always put the heaviest, uncrushable things—shoes, books if you're taking any—on the bottom. Slip shoes into a plastic bag to prevent them from soiling your clothes. Put bras and panties in another plastic bag so they're easy to find and remove without tearing through everything else in the valise. Fold and wrap in tissue large and/or crushable items.

A few years ago I bought three black cases—the kind that salesmen use to carry samples from place to place. These cases come in several sizes. The size I bought is just long enough so that a street-length dress can be packed inside, full-length, without folding. (Evening gowns need to be folded over near the bottom of the skirt.) I take two of these cases with me when I'm going to be away from home for several weeks and need to take a lot of clothes to see me through a variety of circumstances in different kinds of climates. In one case I pack only warm-weather clothes. Cold-weather clothes have a separate case of their own. The great thing about traveling with these cases is that because of their size, dresses, suits, coats, etc., can be packed flat (I hang them on hangers first) and stay virtually wrinkle-free until I need them—which could be weeks after I leave home. In fact, when I'm in a cold-weather place I don't even bother to open and unpack the warm-weather clothes.

House Guesting: Your Place and Theirs

When people come to stay with you for a weekend or a week, you want them to have a good time. You also want them to feel comfortable and at home in your home.

One of the ways you can make sure their stay with you is enjoyable is to find out—before they come—what kind of things they'd like to do as your guest. If you're a New Yorker, you may want to make arrangements for them to see a Broadway show or two, or take them to the Metropolitan Opera or the ballet. If you live in the country, you may want to show your guests the various points of local interest. Or, depending on where you live and the time of year, you may be determined that they get their fill of sunning, swimming, skiing, tennis playing, etc. You'll also want to include them in any social plans you've made and perhaps plan a party or two (or more) of your own during their visit. In fact, you may have the impulse to schedule each and every moment of your guests' stay. Don't. Or at least don't until you've checked with them first.

Maybe your guests would really prefer a relaxed, unhurried time spent with you and your family. (I know that very often that's exactly what *I* want when I go to visit at the homes of friends.)

The good hostess is aware that some of her guests may want to take things easy—at least some of the time—and allows them to do just that. If she has social obligations that must be met, she gives her guests the option of joining her or not. She does not expect that her guests will always want to tag along while she runs errands, shops, picks the children up from school. In other words, a good hostess provides for her guests' enjoyment but at the same time lets them live at their own pace.

Small touches also go a long way toward making a guest feel comfortable and welcome. Fresh flowers and a bowl of fruit in the guest room. Perhaps a pretty pitcher kept filled with ice water. A terry cloth robe hung behind the door. One or two novels and a selection of current magazines on a table near the bed. A good reading lamp. Stationery and postcards in a drawer. An alarm clock. And in the guest bathroom, a hair dryer and magnifying mirror. All the comforts of home away from home.

So much for the good hostess. What about the good guest?

The important thing is to treat your hostess's possessions with at least as much care as you would your own. This is another one of those suggestions that seem almost too obvious to mention and yet we've all heard stories about guests who splash from the pool to the living room, dripping water onto fresh-waxed parquet floors, flopping into expensively upholstered chairs and sofas in soaking-wet bathing suits. Guests who play records and then leave them out of their jackets, scattered across the floor. Guests who borrow cars with full tanks and return them with the gas indicator registering "empty." Guests who borrow horses and then race them till they're ready to drop. And perhaps worst of all, guests who are charming and amiable to all the grown-ups but ignore (or treat as nuisances) the children of the host and hostess.

The guest who gets invited back, obviously, is the guest who never loses sight of the fact that she's staying in someone's home—not a hotel—and that her host and hostess are just that, not innkeepers. As much as possible, she does things for herself rather than sitting back and waiting for someone to do them for her. She doesn't disappear for hours on end only to reappear just as dinner is being served. She offers to help with meals. She takes an interest in the children if there are any.

If there are servants and they've been especially attentive to her needs, she tips them. (It's always better to do this without saying anything to the host and hostess; they'll only tell you that it isn't necessary. Instead, leave an envelope with a little thank-you note someplace where the maid—or whoever—will find it. Or deliver it in person.)

And of course, as soon as the good guest gets back home again, she writes a thank-you note and sends a gift.

The All-Important Decorator

Can you furnish a house in a lovely, warm, creative way without calling in a decorator to help? Certainly. But be warned. It takes time and a lot of running around and a lot of getting to know what's available and where and for how much. Then, unless you're very handy and you and your husband can do much of the physical work yourselves—painting, papering, upholstering, etc.—it takes dealing with painters and paperhangers and upholsterers, and, well, do-it-yourself decorating is undoubtedly very satisfying, but it is also a long, invariably frustrating undertaking.

My advice to the woman who can afford it is this: find a good decorator and learn how to work with him.

How *do* you find one? Unless you go directly to an established "name" decorator, nothing beats the recommendation of a fully satisfied client. Ask among your friends; ask your friends to ask *their* friends. Magazines such as *House & Garden* and *Architectural Digest* often feature the work of up-and-coming young decorators, some of whom may be located in your area. Many good decorators are in touch with antique and fine-furniture dealers, so you might ask *them* for recommendations. Another possibility is to call the best department store in your area and ask for the names of the decorators who do their model rooms.

Once you have the names of two or three possibilities in hand, you're going to want to see samples of their work. (Most decorators have portfolios of photographs of the rooms, or homes, they've done. You might also want to ask if it would be possible to "tour" the homes of some of the decorator's more recent clients.)

Then sit down and talk. You should be prepared to give the decorator an idea of what you have in mind—your preferences in color, style, design—whether you prefer a clean, modern look or feel more comfortable in a traditional setting. (Incidentally, if you want clean and modern and the decorator's portfolio is heavily weighted in favor of the more elaborate and traditional, he's probably not the man for you. It works the other way around too.)

I always look for a certain "chemistry"—rapport, if you wish—in all my dealings with people. When that chemistry is missing, I never feel entirely happy about entering into an important relationship with that person—and I think a relationship with a decorator is an important one.

That's why when I met Mark Hampton I knew immediately that he was the decorator for me. The rapport was perfect. I remember

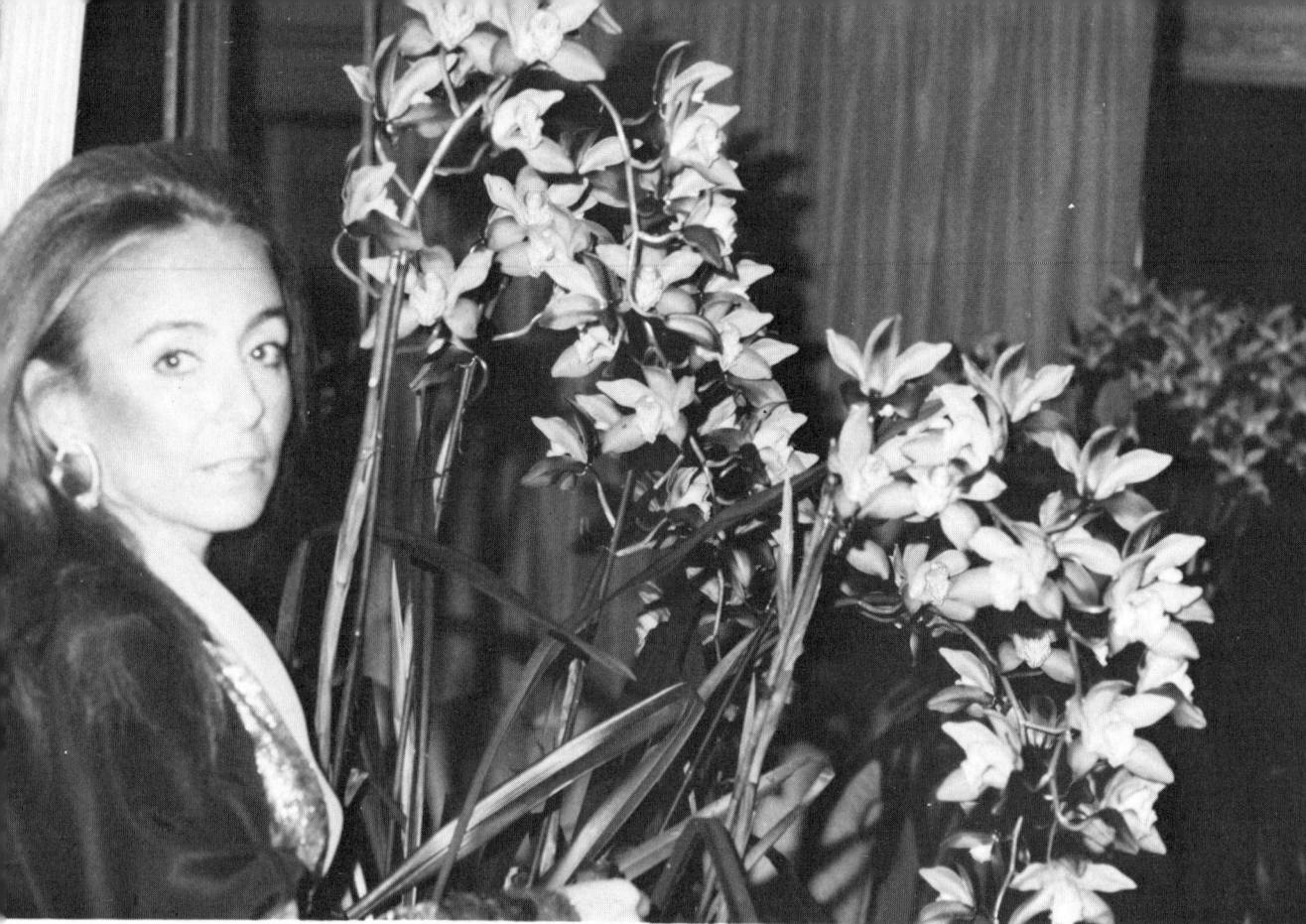

Orchids, my favorite flower, need a great deal of care. As they get taller and heavier, they must be tied together with the twist-type closures that are used for plastic bags. That's what I'm doing here. (PHOTO: LEE GUBER)

talking about redoing one of the rooms in my apartment. Mark asked me what I had in mind and for a moment I couldn't think how to express what I felt the room should be. Then it occurred to me: it should have the easy, lived-in good looks of an old Hermès bag. He knew what I meant the instant the words were out of my mouth. I'm delighted with the results.

Mark also seemed to know, without my having to spell it out in so many words, that I don't like fussy little spindly-legged pieces that look as though they might tip over at the brush of a skirt. That I like to put my feet up on a table without worrying that it's going to collapse. That I wanted a house that is elegant but comfortable, pretty but not dainty, feminine but not cute. We worked it out together and I love my house.

If you have no idea of what you want, then you may as well put yourself entirely in the hands of your decorator and let him make all the decisions. I've known people who left the city for the summer, leaving instructions with their decorator to do anything, but have it done by the time they came back in September. Sometimes it works out very nicely.

I prefer to be involved every step of the way. I give Mark a general idea of what I want. Then he goes out to scout the market for samples. When he's collected five or six "possibles," he either has them delivered to the house (as in the case of wallpaper or other easily portable objects), or together we go out and take a look at them. He understands me well enough by now to know that when I see some-

Mark Hampton did this room for me: off-white walls, rattan furniture, natural straw floor covering. It's a room after my favorite song: "A room without windows, a room without doors, no bells ringing, no telephone." I call it my padded cell.

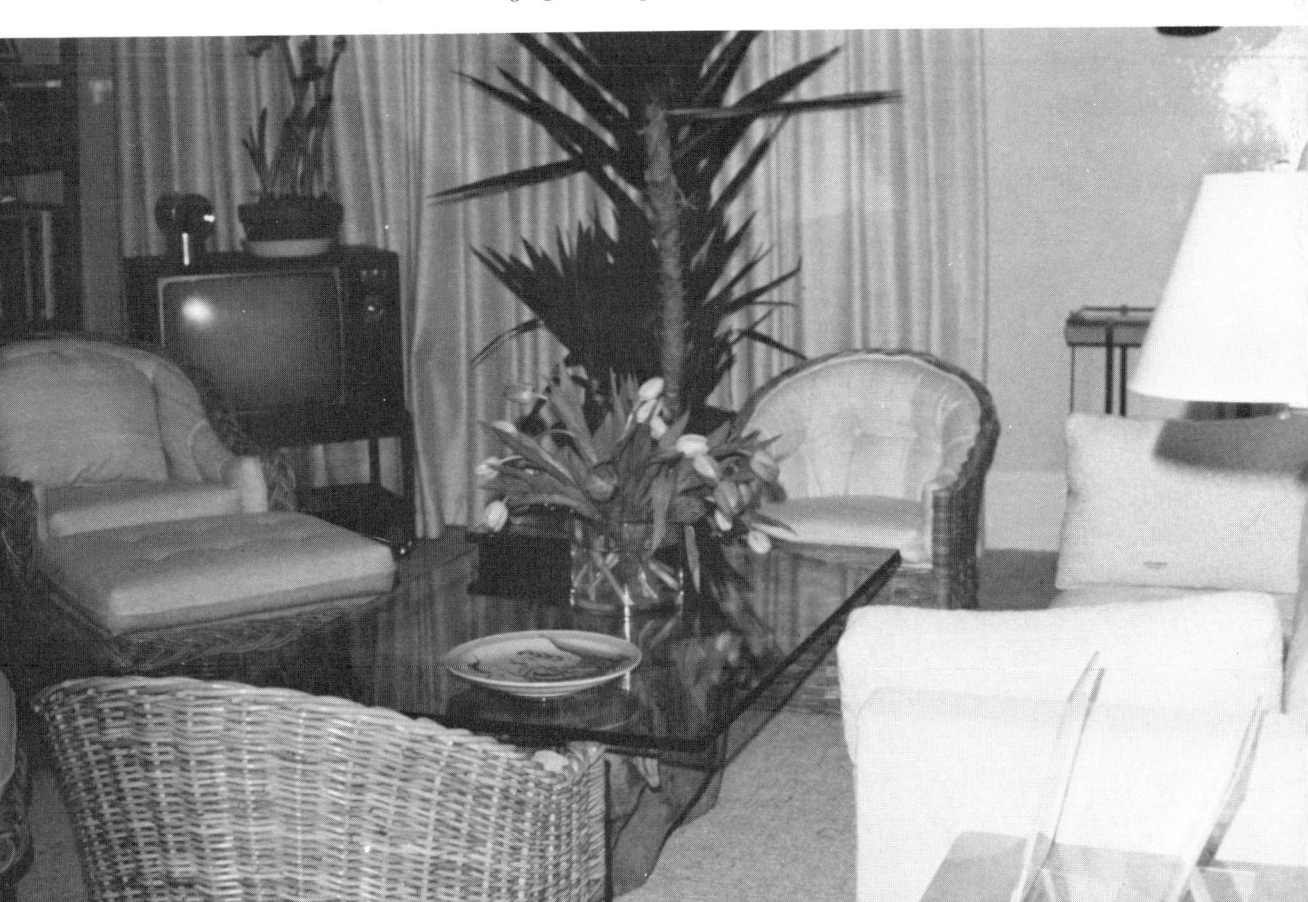

thing, and I brighten up and say "yes" immediately, then "yes" it is. (I hardly ever change my mind when my first impressions are so positive.) "No" is no. And "well, maybe" is also "no."

You may need more time to think things over, and you should have it. But decorator or not, don't allow yourself to be talked into buying

For relaxation I read or do needlepoint. This is one panel of a four-panel needlepoint screen that covers a whole wall in my entrance hall—one my larger projects, and, maybe the reason I wear glasses now. (PHOTO: LEE GUBER)

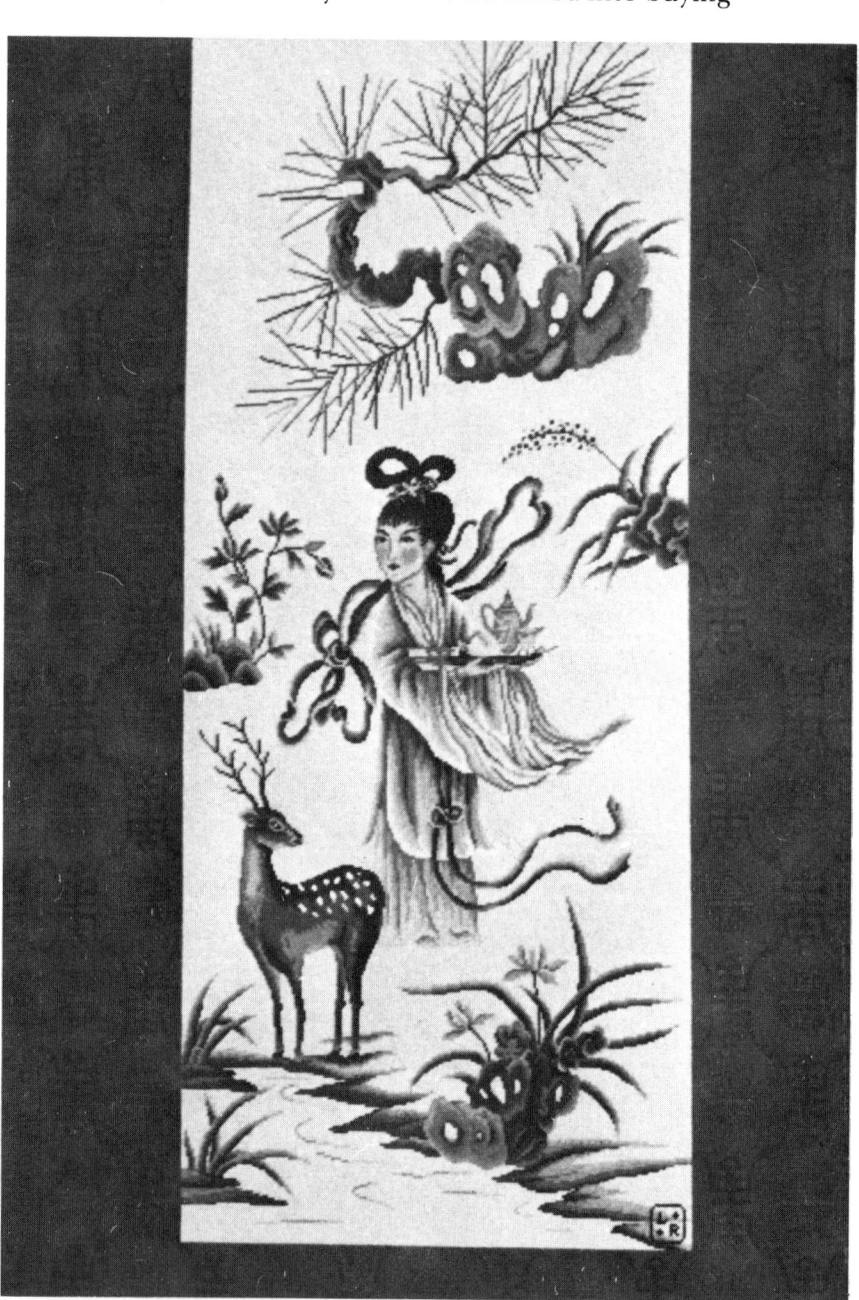

a color scheme, or a design, or even an ashtray that isn't compatible with your personal style. As I've mentioned many times in this book, *you* are the one who has to live with it.

Charity Begins at . . .

Charity work isn't necessarily a part of living with style. You could give money instead. In fact, every once in a while someone asks me, "Why do you run yourself ragged for this charity or that charity? Why don't you just write out a check and be done with it?"

Sometimes I ask myself that same question. I can and do give money to certain charities, and I feel better for having done it. But I want to do more—much more—for the charities that I care most deeply about—those that help children. United Cerebral Palsy (I worked on a telethon, answering phones, taking pledges, for eighteen hours straight). Lenox Hill Hospital (as chairman of their first dinner dance I helped raise $300,000; as ticket co-chairman for the 1977 benefit, I helped raise $1,000,000).

Since collecting money is a primary function of any charity, I try to involve myself directly in the money-raising process. Anyone who's ever done it knows: raising money for charity can be as demanding and time-consuming as a full-time job. Only you don't get paid in dollars and cents; you do get the feeling of having contributed something of yourself to a cause you believe in. That's why I do it.

Becoming involved in a charity is a great way to meet people. There are the luncheon meetings, the teas, and the gala benefit balls. If I were new to the city and didn't know a soul, perhaps I'd pick a charity and go to all the luncheons and teas with an eye to broadening my range of acquaintances. Many women do it, and I think it's marvelous that they're able to accomplish good works at the same time that they're establishing social contacts.

As chairman of two or three fund-raising projects, I learned, for example, that the people you work with are crucial. When you're new to charity work it may come as a rude awakening to discover that many, many people lend their names to a cause, and even attend a few meetings, but when it's time to deliver—do the work—they don't. However, there are always some few people who *are* there to work. I know, for instance, that when my friend Marilyn Evins is on a committee, she gives her all. It is not in her to do anything else. I almost always turn to her for help when I need it. The same is true of Phyllis Wagner. It works both ways: when either of them needs me, I'm there.

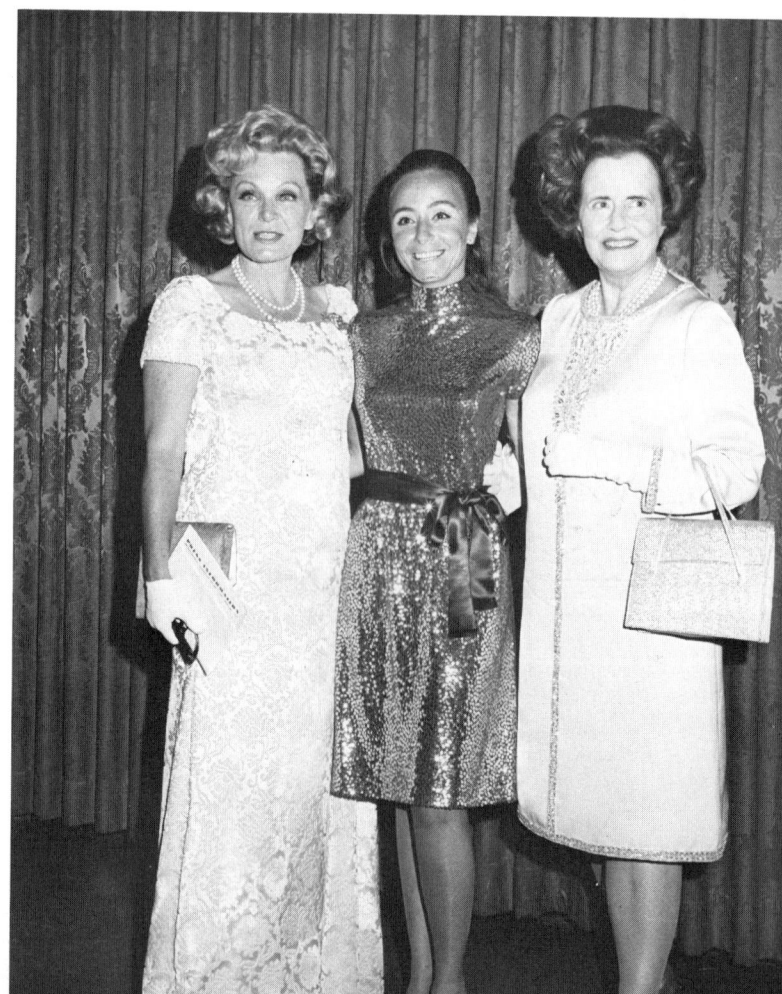

As chairwoman of a theater party to benefit United Cerebal Palsy in 1966, I worked with Jane Pickens Langley (left) and Mary Lasker. (PHOTO: ED SULLIVAN)

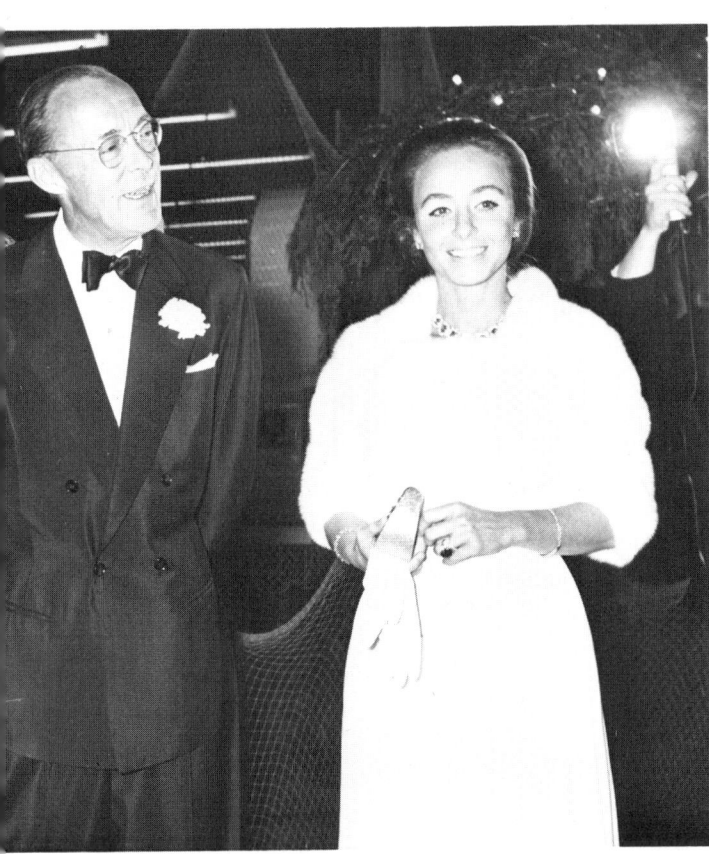

With Prince Bernhard of the Netherlands at a 1966 benefit for the American Cancer Society. (PHOTO: WAGNER INTERNATIONAL PHOTO)

At the Red Cross Ball in Palm Beach with Marjorie Merriweather Post.

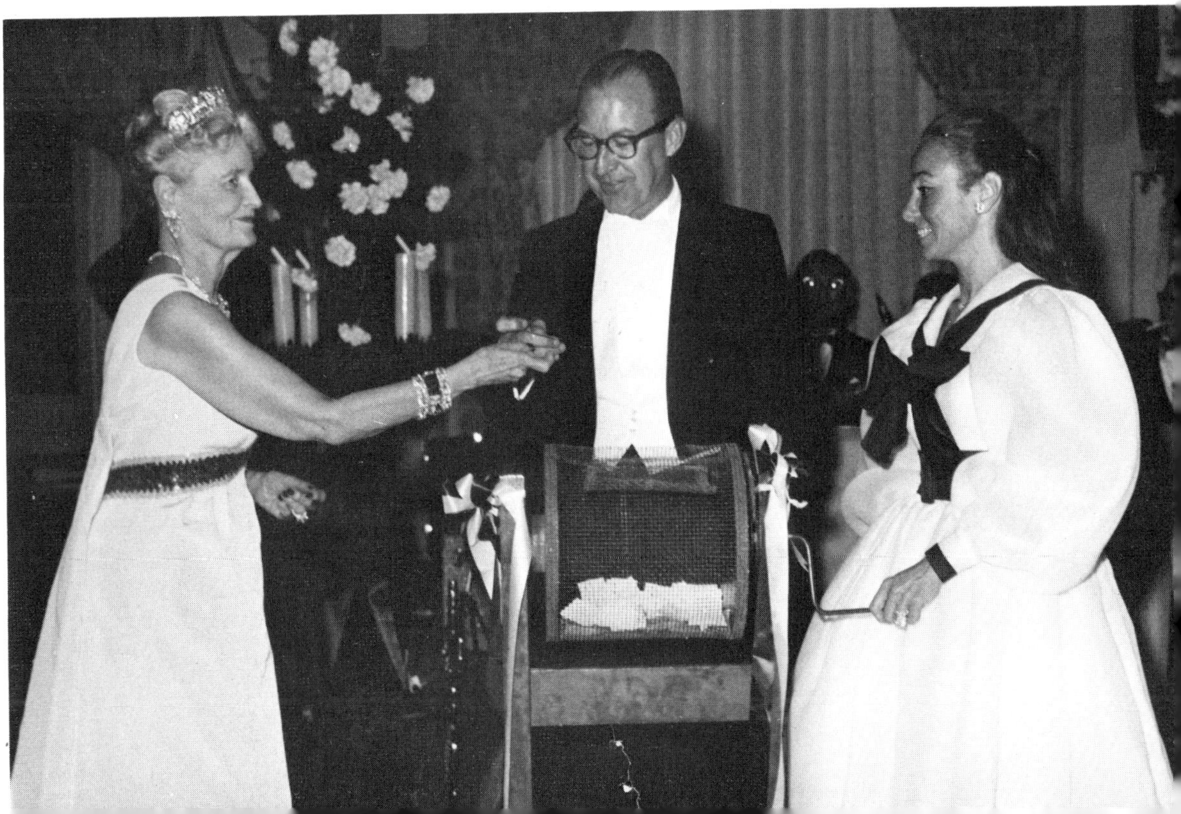

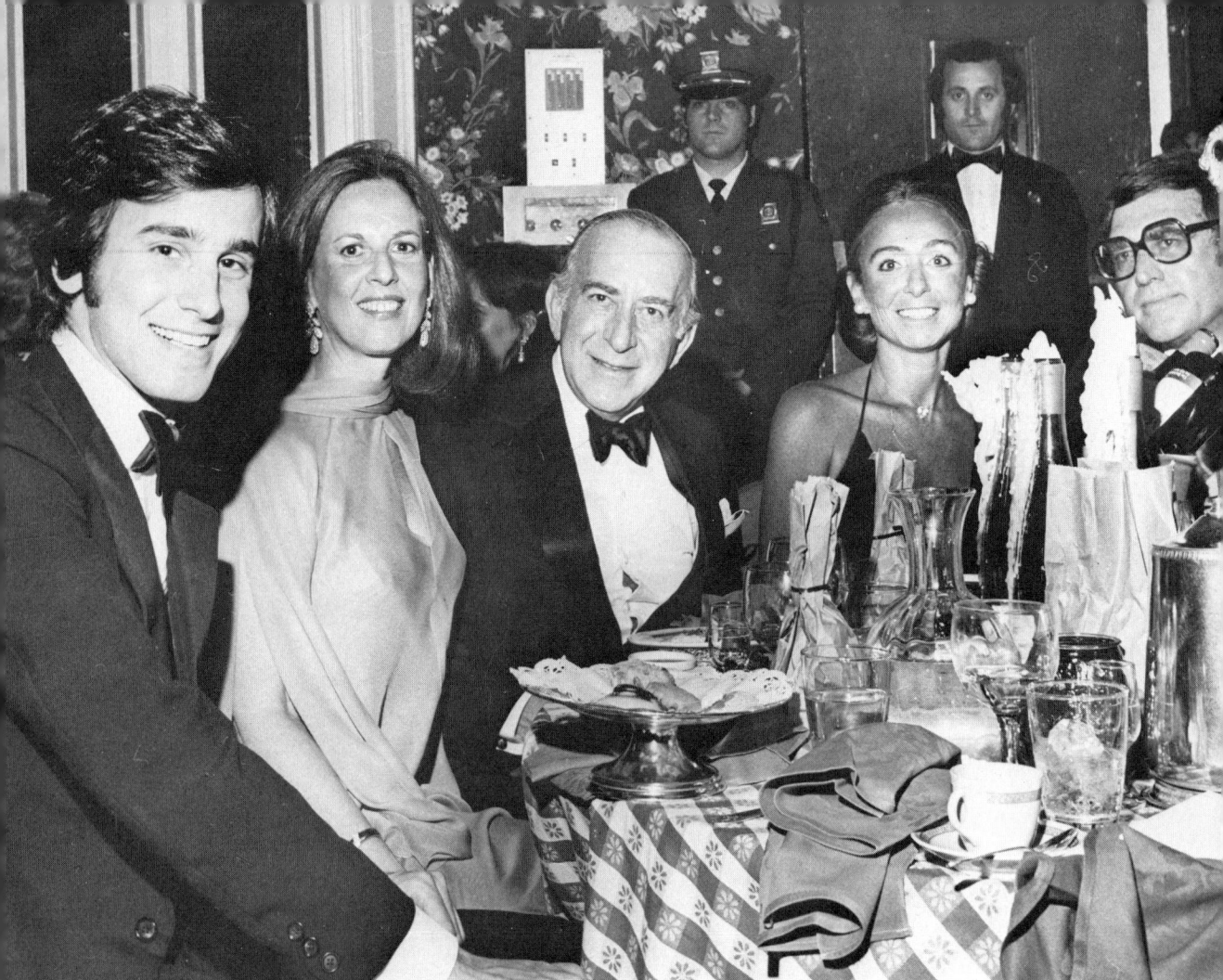

At the Lenox Hill Hospital benefit in 1977. From the left: my son Jeffrey, Mrs. Saklad and Dr. Maurice Saklad, me, and Lee Guber. (PHOTO: BILL MARK)

Even with the best people in the world working at your side, it's still far from easy to raise money. Everyone gets "hit" so many times for contributions, and no one can be expected to give to everything. The people who are hit hardest and most often are the people with the most money. As a result, many of them are also the most reluctant to give. (Not that they don't give at all, mind you; only that many of them give very generously to two or three pet charities and little or nothing to others.)

For this reason, it may be a good idea to try to find out who gives to what. Keep in mind that if someone gave generously last year (often, records are kept), they're the ones to go after again this year. There's a certain reciprocity at work, too. If I've donated to a certain person's charity, I may be especially persistent in asking that same person to donate to mine. (When you're getting nowhere, thank the person nicely, tell him or her you've enjoyed your little talk, and put an end to it.) I also try to ask for money only from the people who have already asked me. That may sound as though I'm limiting the phone calls I can make, but believe me, I'm not. There are dozens and dozens, maybe hundreds, who fall into this category.

One of the hardest things to decide on when you're working on a charity fund-raiser is what to charge for a ticket. I tend to take a very hard line: charge whatever you can. Get whatever you can get. Don't worry about what you'll have to charge next year if you charge a great deal this year. The time is now and the job is to raise as much money as possible. As someone I know says, "Lightning only strikes once." And as someone else I know says, "I'm not in this thing for the finger sandwiches."

Charity work isn't all work and no fun. Last year at the Waldorf, a "Cooking Gala" was held to benefit the March of Dimes. About twenty people were invited to cook their favorite dishes right there in the main ballroom in front of thousands of seated onlookers. The Waldorf chefs knew in advance what the "celebrity cooks" (as they were called) would be concocting and approximations of those dishes were served to the people seated at tables who were in effect the audience. The cooking gala was really a contest; eighteen prizes were offered. Lee Guber and I cooked chicken capriccioso, and though I always play to win, we didn't win this one. Novelist and food writer Gael Greene placed first with her duck with grapes. But as they say, it was all for a good cause.

By now, many people don't get excited about charity balls anymore, but a cooking contest is something different. Keep it in mind if you're ever stumped for fund-raising ideas.

6

My Favorite People, Places, and Things

I'd like to share with you some one-of-a-kind people, places, and experiences that have had great impact on my life and my style.

Motherhood

First with me is being a mother, raising my children, and now seeing what fine, healthy, good young people they are. That's the one-of-a-kind experience of a lifetime. If I sound like a doting mother, well, it's true, I am. They're attractive, unspoiled people. Their feet are on the ground, and they are contributing members of society.

Steven, my eldest, is twenty-seven. He's funny, gregarious, and charming. Jeffrey is gentle, introspective, and enormously creative. Susan is sensitive and modest, and shares with me a love of children.

I put a lot into them but I got—I'm still getting—a lot out of them too. I wish I knew how many times I've said to them, singly or all together, "I don't care what other children do or are allowed to do, I only care about what *you* do." I said "no" to them often. "No," I think, is very hard to say to one's children. To take the responsibility of saying "no," and then standing by your "no," to try to be the Rock of Gibraltar and not crumble—it is very difficult indeed. It's much easier to say "yes," "go ahead," "do what you please," "I don't care." I wasn't permissive. It was always discipline with a lot of love. I'm very pleased with the results.

A year ago I wrote them each a letter. I told them that no matter how they chose to live their lives, earn their livings, they were to do it for themselves, to make themselves happy, not for me.

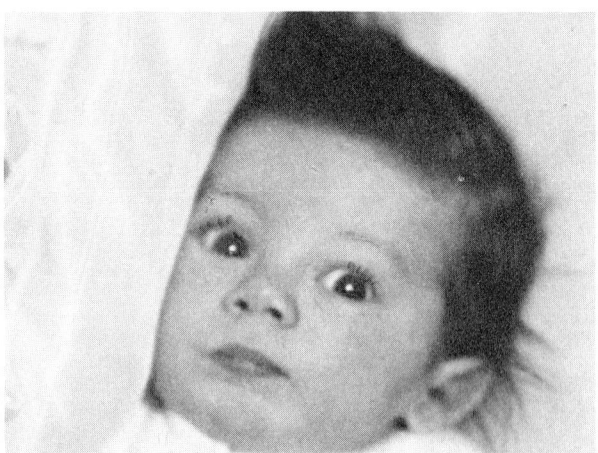

My brood as babies: Steven at one month

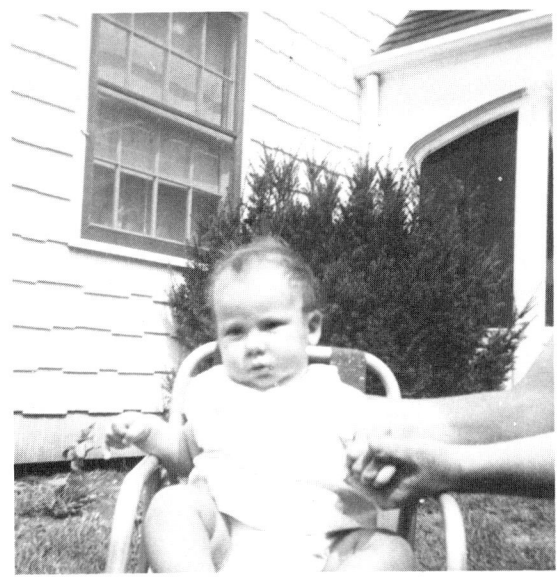

Jeffrey at two months

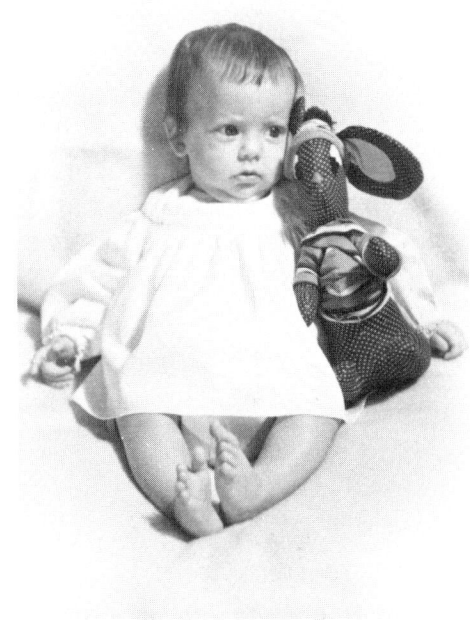

and Susan at one month.

Places and Things

VENICE: My favorite city and absolutely the most romantic place I've ever visited. Breathtakingly beautiful, Venice is a city to come back to over and over again.

Everyone knows about the Canals of Venice but hearing about them or looking at pictures doesn't prepare you for the surprise of actually seeing the watery streets, the gondolas with their uniformed "chauffeurs" parked in front of the hotels and townhouses, the delivery boats filled with flowers and produce, the police boats, the ambulance boats, the underwater cemetery. It is the most astonishing city in the world.

In Venice I stay at the Gritti Palace, a very small, beautiful old hotel where the service is perfect. Another good hotel, about 30 minutes by boat from St. Mark's Square and the Gritti, is the Lido at Lido Beach. The Lido is as gigantic as the Gritti is small and used to be famous for its casino.

Venice is an hour or less by plane from Rome or Milan. Unless you know for sure you'll be going to a ball or other gala evening party, you needn't take an evening gown. Pants, jeans, and for dressy evenings, a simple long T-shirt dress or evening pajamas will see you through.

The tourist sights are spectacular—do not miss the ducal palace, the Accademia, and the Ca D'Oro; spend as much time as you can walking through this magical city. Remember to have dinner at least once at Harry's Bar, and be sure to visit Martini's, where they have the biggest shrimp in the world. I always try to visit the ducal palace

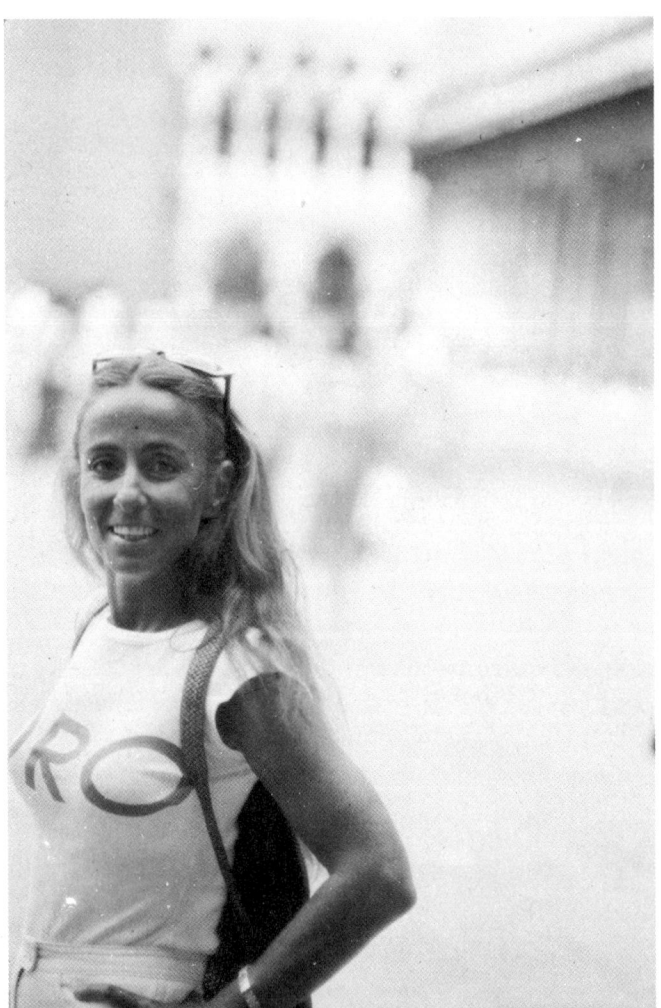

In Venice: Strolling in St. Mark's Square (my shirt says *oro*—Italian for gold);

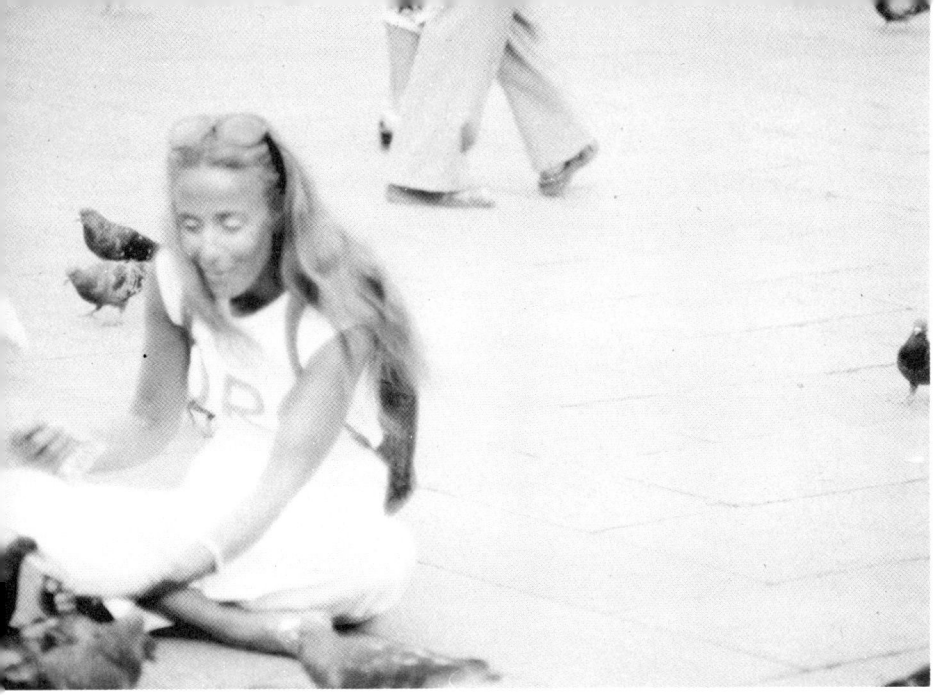

feeding the pigeons;

and time out in a garden restaurant. (PHOTO: LEE GUBER)

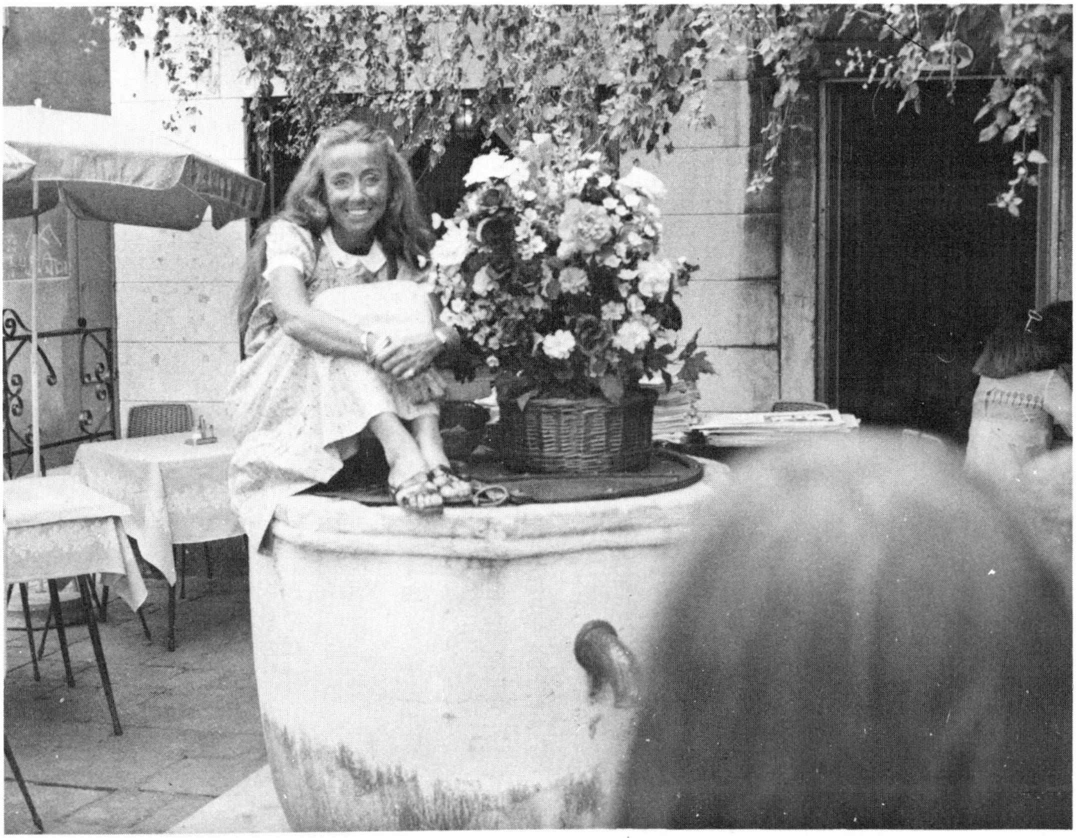

and all of St. Mark's Square, as well as the glass factory at Murano to see chandeliers and other decorative glass objects in the making.

ISRAEL: If Venice is my favorite city, Israel is the country I like best to visit. I've traveled there at least once a year for the last nine or ten years. Like Venice, I can't get enough of it.

Israel, though, is a very different kind of trip and calls up different emotions. Israel fills me with pride. But even if I weren't Jewish, I know Israel would affect me; it is such a moving testament to human strength, courage, and ingenuity. It is all true: the Israelis *have* made the desert bloom and forged thriving, productive modern cities alongside ancient reminders of the past.

With Merle Oberon, Jerome Zipkin, and Audrey and George Zauderer, I had the opportunity to visit Israel just a few months after the Six-Day War. At that time we met Meyer Weisgal, head of the famed Weizmann Institute of Science in Rehovot, and Ezer Weizmann, who was commander-in-chief of Israeli defense forces during the war. Both gentlemen told us of their experiences during the conflict, and Weisgal took us to the Golan Heights where we saw Russian tanks, abandoned but still poised atop the hills—just as they were only months before when so many Israeli troops died in the attempt to stem their advance.

In Israel, I'm up and out by seven and spend all day every day discovering new sights and visiting old ones over and over again. Not to miss: the Chagall windows and the Dead Sea Scrolls in Jerusalem. The Wailing Wall. The Sinai desert. A kibbutz. The winding back streets of Tel Aviv and Jerusalem. (In a little shop on one of those back streets, I found a strikingly beautiful necklace of ceramic beads, each shaped like an ankh—the symbol that became such a popular jewelry item after it appeared on the cover of Jacqueline Susann's best-selling novel *The Love Machine*. As it turned out, the necklace, which I bought, was made about 300 B.C.)

In Israel, dress for comfort. Wear a T-shirt and pants, jeans, or a skirt in a sturdy fabric for sightseeing. Low-heeled walking shoes are a must. At night, slip into something simple: a short or long T-shirt dress is perfect.

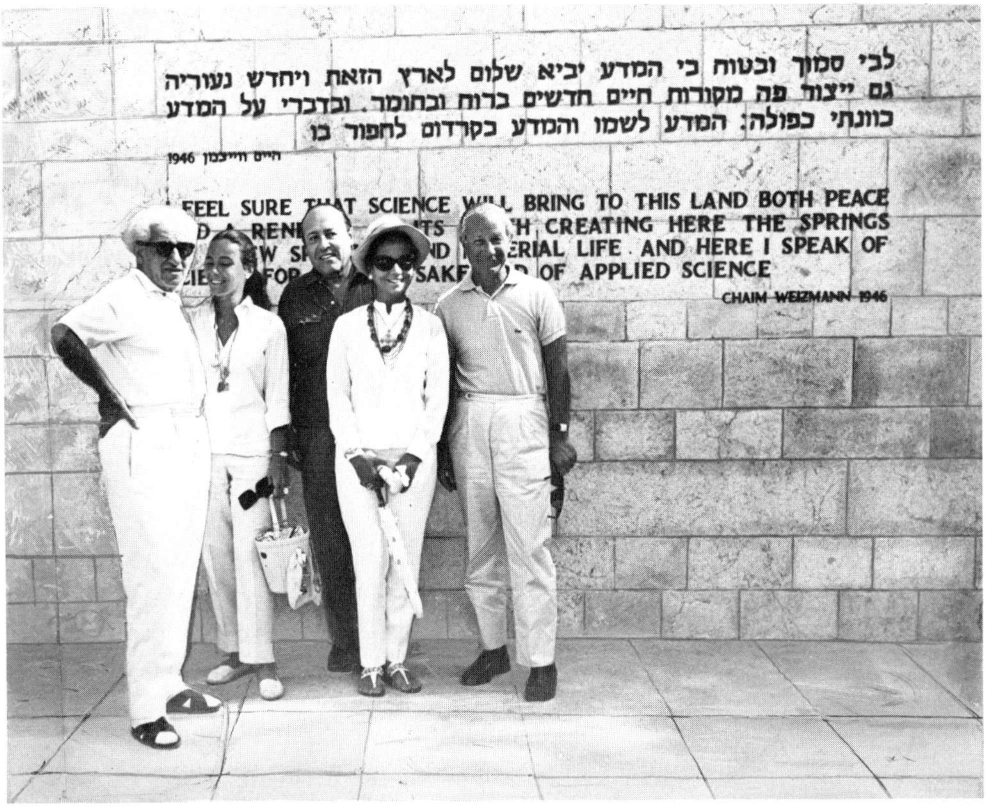

Outside the Weizmann Institute in Rehovoth, Israel, with Meyer Weisgal, Jerome Zipkin, Merle Oberon, and Dr. Alfred Steiner. At right, on a tour of the Institute with Meyer Weisgal. (PHOTO: BEN-ZVI)

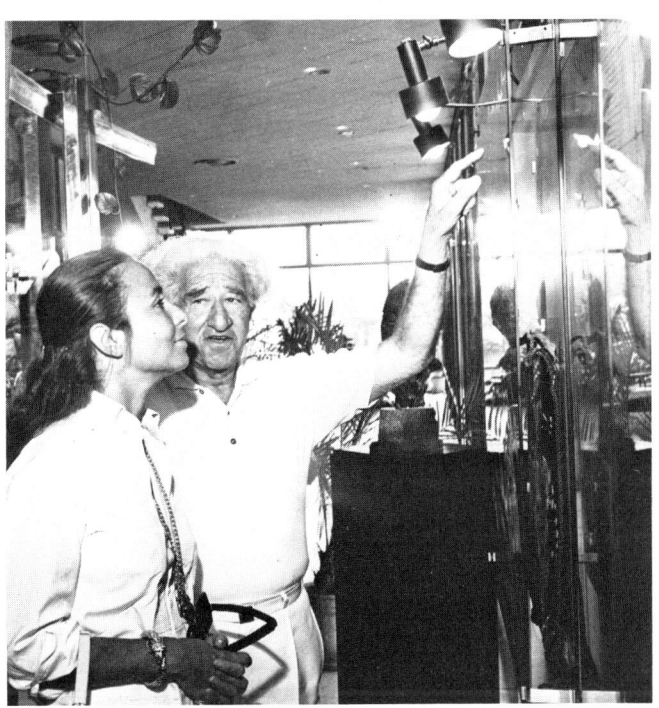

PALM SPRINGS: If I were to buy a house, I'd buy one in this hot, dry, but marvelously lush California desert community where day after day I can bake to my favorite shade of tan (comfortably, because of the low humidity). At night the mercury drops to 50 or so; perfect sleeping weather.

The Ingleside Inn is a good place to stay. A very large old home converted into a hotel, everything about it is charming: the furniture (all antiques), the food, and the service.

For me, the only thing better than staying at the Ingleside Inn is staying with my friends Mr. and Mrs. Daniel Schwartz. Natalie Schwartz is a marvelous hostess. Her house is delightful. Her chef turns out magnificent meals. Her dinner parties are perfection. Her tennis courts superb. Even her pets seem special. Maybe just as important, she seems to know instinctively when and how to leave her guests alone without abandoning them. I'm often tired when I go there to visit, and it shows. The Schwartzes don't insist that I accompany them every place they go while I'm with them; in fact, they don't insist that I do much of anything except take it easy. By the time I get

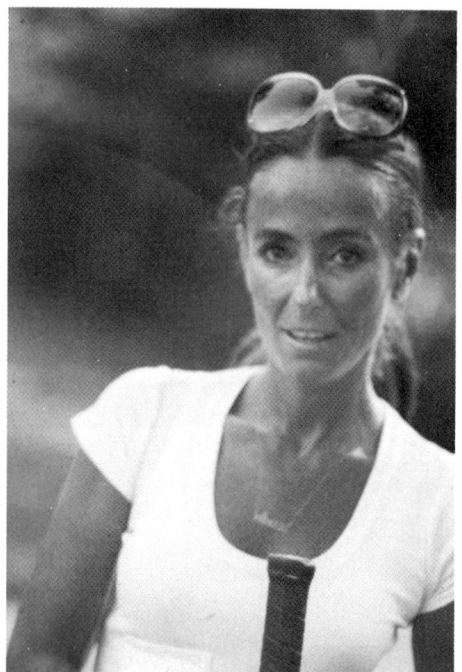

In Palm Springs. I play tennis every chance I get. (PHOTO: LEE GUBER)

back to New York, I'm looking and feeling ten years younger.

PARIS, LONDON, ROME: What can anyone say about them—good or bad—that hasn't been said a thousand times before? They are still the crown jewels (along with New York, I want to add) of Western civilization.

In Paris I stay at the Plaza Athénée, still the ultimate in luxury and service (though I never cease to be amazed at how small are the rooms in even the grandest Paris hotels). For dining out, I adore Le Grand Véfour, Maxim's, and the Relais Plaza.

Just as much fun, for me at any rate, are the informal bistros. On a recent trip I was taken to a marvelous out-of-the-way place called Nos Ancêtres Les Gaulois. Our meal began with a huge basket full of the biggest, ripest, most beautiful raw vegetables imaginable. We were given a pitcher and helped ourselves to wine from a barrel. There was a buffet table of relishes and appetizers, and the entrée was served by a waiter. This delightful, cozy restaurant is on the rue Saint-Louis en l'Isle.

Another highlight of my last trip to Paris was the new Beaubourg Center, which from the outside looks like a child's red and blue Tinkertoy creation.

In London I have stayed at the Connaught and eaten there as well. I have also stayed at Claridge's. They are both first-rate hotels.

When I'm in London I go to the theater as often as I can. A visit to London wouldn't be complete without spending at least part of a Sunday afternoon strolling through Hyde Park and listening to the soapbox orators. There are dozens of them, in all kinds of weather, poised on their wooden crates, holding forth on just about every subject under the sun.

New in London—at least since I was last there—is the beautiful Hayward Gallery, which is located in the South Bank Art Centre along with the National Theatre. Also new is a fabulous pizza parlor called Pizzaland. It is decorated with fresh and attractive green-and-white tilework, and pizza addicts like myself behave like they're in a three-star Michelin restaurant.

Rome is another one of those "addictive" cities that I feel I must go back to over and over again. (But then I've always been drawn to

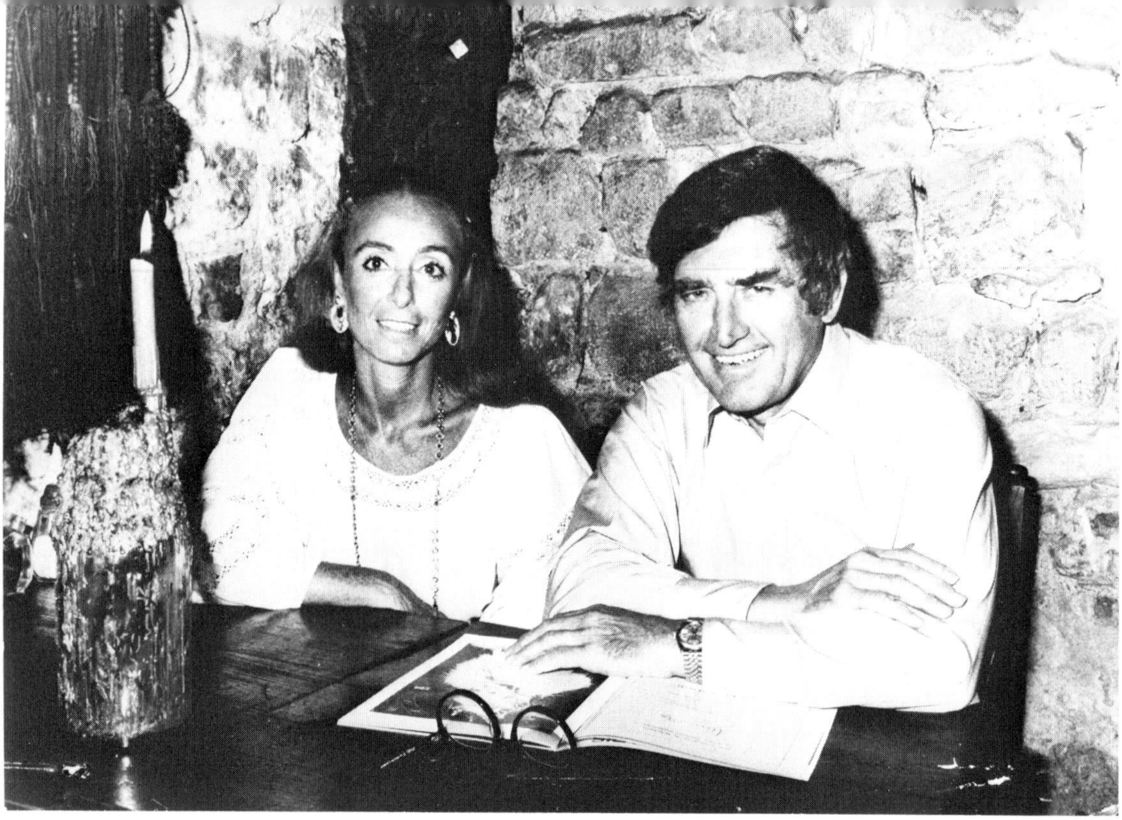

In Paris with Lee Guber at one of our extraordinary restaurant "finds": Nos Ancêtres Les Gaulois. (PHOTO: LEE GUBER)

Soapbox orators are the major entertainment in London's Hyde Park on a Sunday afternoon. (PHOTO: LEE GUBER)

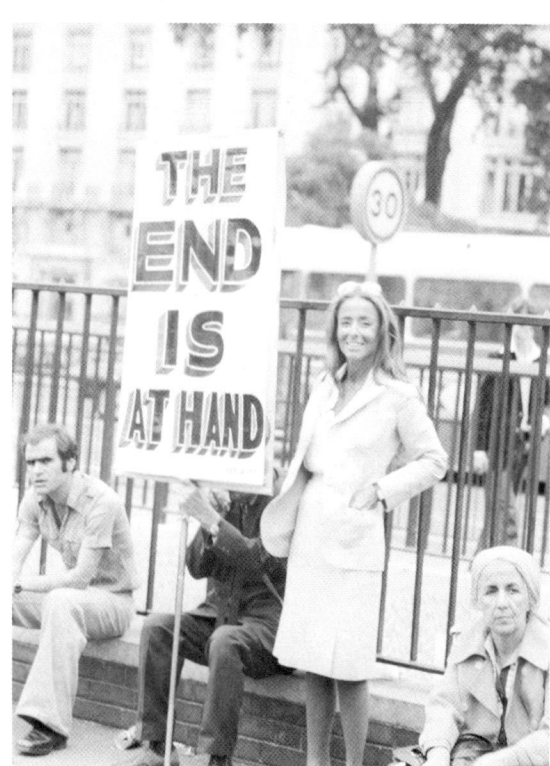

all things Italian.) In Rome I throw three coins in every fountain I pass (and there are hundreds), see the Vatican, and gawk and gawk at the Sistine Chapel.

The Grand Hotel in Rome, where I stayed once with Bern and Billy Rose, has beyond a doubt the largest, grandest, most luxurious suites I've ever seen.

Italian food is my kind of food—even bad Italian food. So it's almost impossible for me to single out a favorite restaurant in Rome; in a pinch I guess I'd choose the beautiful Hosteria Dell'Orso, though there are a couple of restaurants on the very beautiful Piazza Navonna that run it a close second.

NEW YORK: It's my hometown and I love it. I've lived here all my life and though I love to go away, I love coming back almost as much. Yes, it's too hot in the summer and too cold in the winter, and parts of it are dirty. Lately it's been a very troubled town. But it's a city with a heart and a soul and a spirit all its own. I'm a New York booster and I'm sure I always will be.

Central Park, the Bronx Zoo, the Village, SoHo (which I'm only just now discovering), the Broadway shows, the ballet, the museums. They never cease to delight.

As for the Statue of Liberty—well, I'm ashamed to say that like many native New Yorkers, I never paid much attention to it until recently. And then I decided to take a closer look.

It's magnificent. The boat that takes you to the statue is packed with people, all kinds, young people, old people, black people, yellow people, white people, well dressed and poorly dressed and everything in between. The statue is awe-inspiring because of its size and what it means (or meant, or should mean). There's a little museum at its base, and a gift shop with souvenirs and trinkets for sale, and a restaurant selling hamburgers and hot dogs.

Inside the statue is a spiral staircase. Climb high enough and you can look out the windows set in Liberty's crown. Climb higher still and you can stand inside the torch. I didn't quite make it to her shoulders, but I'll try harder next time because I'm going back soon.

NEW YORK RESTAURANTS: Part of the fun of being a New Yorker is having so many great restaurants so close at hand. Everyone has favorites. Here are some of mine:

Alfredo's. Alfredo Viazzi has several restaurants. The one I like best is the first, the Trattoria on Bank Street. Try the stuffed mushrooms; any of the pasta dishes; the asparagus wrapped in prosciutto that you can dip in pesto sauce; and the marvelous platters of just-cooked vegetables, a slice of sausage, and a piquant green sauce for dipping.

Pearl's. It's one of the best Chinese places in town. I always have the lettuce wrapped around a mysterious filling, then dipped in a rich plum sauce. Then rice pancakes; baby spare ribs; clams in black bean sauce; maybe beef cooked with broccoli and ginger; or beef with red and green peppers. After that they have to carry me home.

Orsini's. It's all sunshine, plants, and beautiful tilework. I especially enjoy going there because Orsini is a friend of eighteen years or so. Great for lunch or dinner. At lunch, I like melted mozzarella cheese with capers and anchovy sauce and arugala salad. Dinner? Always veal or pasta, or veal *and* pasta.

Elaine's. A great place to sit and watch and be watched. Most people don't go there for the food, but I do. (I also like Elaine.) Try the pimiento and anchovy appetizer. Sometimes I have spaghetti with white clam sauce, and the broiled veal chop.

Twenty-One. I like to sit downstairs in the bar, where the ceiling is hung with dozens of miniature toys—airplanes, trucks, cars—and the tables are covered with red and white checkered tablecloths. For lunch, I like the sunset salad; for dinner, mussels when in season.

McDonald's. Hardly just a New York phenomenon, I know. Still, I like a Big Mac "to go" every once in a while or to eat right there in the restaurant. Sometimes nothing but a Big Mac will do.

(Incidentally, on the subject of restaurants, I'm always amused when I hear people fussing about getting the "best" table. And they *do* fuss about it. In case the concept is unknown to you, there are "good" and "bad" tables in many of the world's great restaurants. The food is the same and the prices are the same, no matter where one sits, but the "important" people get the "good" tables—often actually very bad in the sense that they may be in the very middle of a room where traffic is heaviest and a private conversation is almost impossible—while lesser people are banished to "Siberia." In truth, it's not the table that makes a person important; it's the person who makes the table important. So it doesn't matter where you sit. Wherever it happens to be, it's the best table in the room—if you feel that way about it.

One more thing about restaurants: Over the years I've come to realize more and more that one doesn't always have the most marvelous time in the most famous or glamorous or expensive restaurant. Not that I don't appreciate fine food, excellent service, and a charming decor—because I do. But even more important to me is enjoying an evening with people I care about. La Côte Basque or Joe's Diner —when I'm with someone who means something to me, it hardly matters which it is.

THE TALL SHIPS: July 4, 1976, and the Bicentennial celebration. I was lucky enough to have a ringside seat on the aircraft carrier *Forrestal* as the hundreds of tall-masted sailing ships from many foreign countries breezed by, sailors at attention, sails whipped by a fresh wind. A majestic sight, and so was the *Forrestal* itself, the largest U.S. aircraft carrier in service now. A glorious day for our country. (And for me.)

COOKING: Who'd have thought that I'd ever love it? Or do it, not because I have to but because I want to. Not that I didn't know how to broil a lamb chop before, or boil spaghetti in a pot. But that I, who love Nathan's hot dogs and licorice and pizza and hamburger-joint hamburgers, should now be spending hours at the stove, clarifying butter, sautéeing shallots, perfecting my crepe technique! I surprise myself.

My friend Lee Guber was my inspiration. A marvelous cook, taught by Jim Beard, he's doing his best to teach me everything he knows. I've learned how to read—really read—a recipe. Now I know the difference between whipping and stirring, folding and beating. I know about all the different kinds of knives and why some pans are better than others for certain things. I'm even overcoming an aversion to eggs. If I can just learn to think of "omelettes" instead of soft-boiled eggs, I'll be all right.

Sunday night cooking has become a ritual. On Saturday, we pull

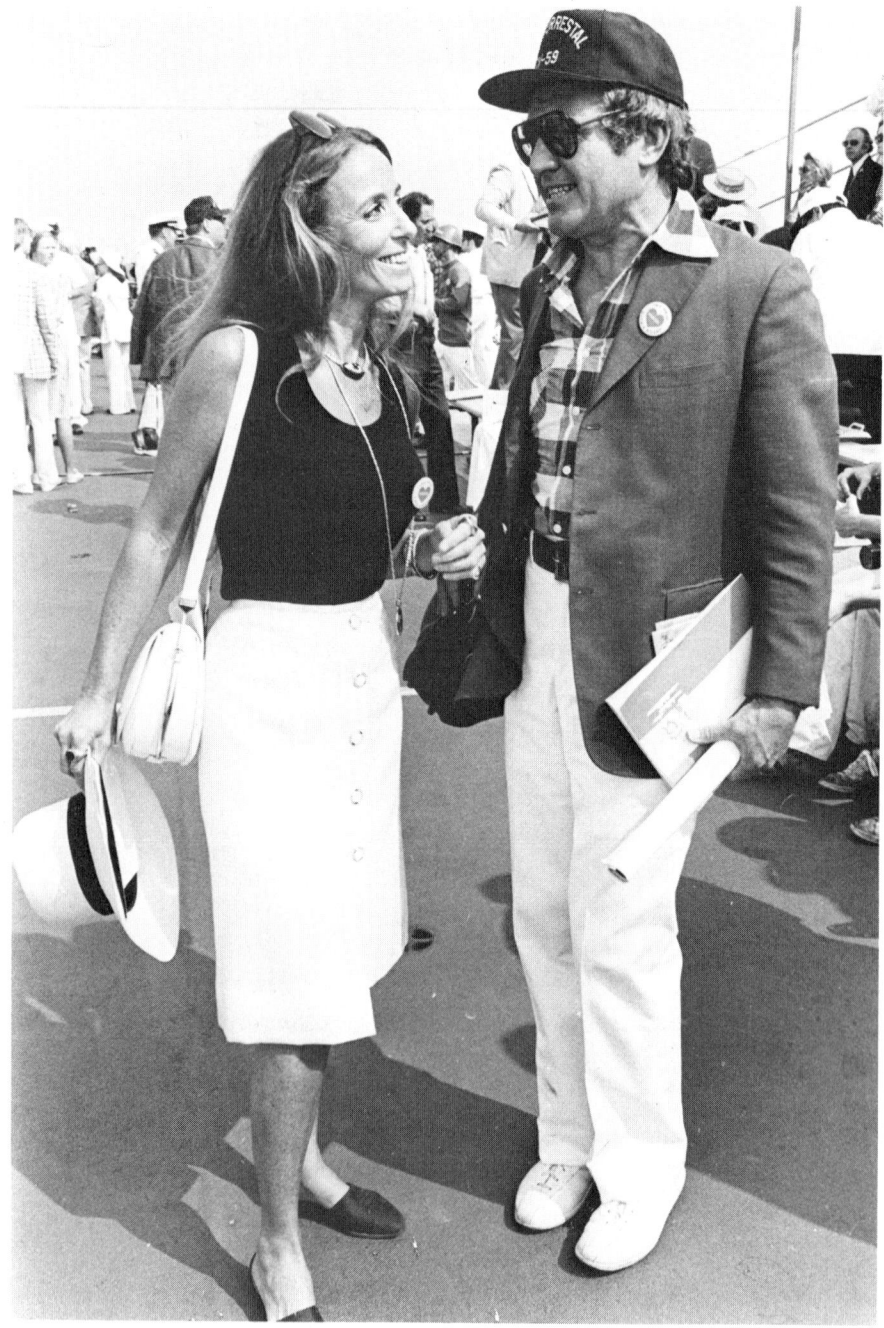

July 4, 1977 on the U.S.S. *Forrestal:* Lee Guber and I had a sensational day watching the procession of tall ships. (PHOTO: WWD)

out the cookbooks and all the folders of recipes saved from *The New York Times*. We plan something interesting, unusual, time-consuming, and a challenge. Then we shop. On Sunday we chop and peel and slice and braise and brown and bake and boil and finally it's ready to eat.

Afterward, there are the dishes. Sure I hate cleaning up. But I do it, it's such a small price to pay.

As a cook, I was born only about two years ago. But I feel I'm quickly reaching my maturity.

HOUSTON: Houston is the city of the future. Vital, alive, awesomely modern in many respects. Despite the city's twenty-first-century gloss, the people of Houston live graciously, in a style all their own.

My friend Joan Schnitzer, for example. She's another of those great hostesses who don't seem to feel the need to plan every second of my time when I visit. She makes me feel wonderfully at home even as she hurries off to luncheons or to run errands in the city (always giving me the choice of joining her or not, as I please).

One of the things I always want very much to do when I'm in Houston is to visit the NASA headquarters. Joan arranged a tour through Deke Slayton, then the NASA chief, who was kind enough to show us around himself. The highlight is always the hour or so spent going through the NASA museum. While at NASA, Slayton introduced me to the Russian astronauts and I saw a mock-up of the Russian space capsule. It would be a great opportunity missed to go to Houston without visiting the NASA museum—and that goes double for couples traveling with their children.

Heart surgeon Dr. Denton Cooley, a one-of-a-kind man if there ever was one, is another reason I always look forward to visiting Houston. On my last trip, he invited me to watch him operate. There I stood in a glass-walled gallery overlooking the operating theater while Cooley and his team down below went about the business of saving lives. At a point in one operation, Cooley held the patient's pulsing heart in his gloved hand. Cooley's secretary, Kitty, came up several times to ask whether I was all right and to find out whether I'd had enough. But it was hours before I could tear myself from the sight of Cooley and his assistants, all working with the quick sureness of artists, master craftsmen. As I left, I noticed a sign on one of the pale blue operating room walls: "Yesterday is gone, today is here, tomorrow may never come."

Cooley operates from early in the morning to seven or eight o'clock at night. Then he records on tape the details of his day's work. After that he checks on the people he has operated on during the day and visits patients scheduled for the next day's surgery. Yet at about ten o'clock in the evening of the day when I watched him operate, Cooley arrived at a dinner party looking fresher and more animated than many of the nine-to-five businessmen in the group. He talked, he laughed, he joked, he danced. How does he maintain that incredible energy? I suspect that the answer has something to do with loving his work—and that sign on the operating room wall.

CAPE KENNEDY AND THE APOLLO 13 LAUNCH: For years, I'd been following the Apollo space program on TV and in the newspapers, but I'd never seen a launching until the spring of 1968, when I went to Cape Kennedy for the Apollo 13 lift-off. The night before, I had dinner with former astronauts Alan Shepard and Walt Cunningham. I knew then what a kid must feel like when he meets a couple of his baseball idols. Neither Shepard nor Cunningham was going up the next day. But Shepard, who was one of the very first U.S. astronauts, had been selected to go up again at a later date.

Lift-off for Apollo 13 was scheduled for midafternoon the following day. Before the launch we went to take a look at a full-size mock-up of the Apollo capsule. Shepard, Cunningham, and I crawled in. It was tiny, so tiny I couldn't fully extend an arm without bumping either into one of them or the capsule wall.

A few hours later we saw the men being loaded into the van that would take them to the launching site. Still later, we took our places about a mile from the rocket. As the countdown went into its final minute there was a hush, and for a while it seemed as though the only things in the world that mattered were the rocket off in the distance with the afternoon sun glinting off its surface and the three men inside the capsule. Finally, the countdown reached "zero." For a moment, nothing happened. Then flames blossomed out at the base of the rocket and it slowly, slowly lifted, then rose, lazily at first and then faster until it disappeared into the cloudless blue.

There were loud cheers from everyone, and for me, a feeling that somewhere inside something was going to burst—with joy and pride and happiness.

I remember asking Shepard why, after one successful launch, he would want to risk his life and repeat the experience. He looked at me and said, "Remember the way you felt watching that launch . . . well, that's the reason for going up again."

ATLANTIC CITY: Years ago I used to drive down to Atlantic City. In those days it was a thriving resort town with grand hotels, a glorious beach, and, on special days, auctions all up and down the boardwalk where one could bid for fine antique furniture, paintings, silver, and even jewelry. Even then Atlantic City had its honky-tonk side: amusement parks, shooting galleries, pinball parlors, and all those little shops lining the boardwalk selling saltwater taffy, peanut butter made fresh before your eyes, jelly apples, corn on the cob (there was always a big barrel of butter on the counter and you dipped the corn yourself). It was all good fun. Over the years, though, Atlantic City went the way of 42nd Street in New York. Sleaze set in.

Now it looks like a new day is dawning on Atlantic City. With gambling legal, Atlantic City will be the new "in" place—a kind of East Coast Las Vegas, maybe better, if only because of the beach.

Last time I was there I learned that already a few of the big hotel companies are buying up the best of the wonderful old hotels with the idea of refurbishing them. There are also plans to build luxurious new hotels and casinos. It won't be long before smart little gift shops and boutiques will be taking over some of the boarded-up space. Excellent new restaurants will be coming in. The beach will be cleaned up. Watch and see. (I only hope they'll be smart enough to keep the Ferris wheel, the pizza stands, and the shooting galleries.)

DISNEYLAND: I spent only one day in this fabulous place, but I could have stayed weeks, months. I saw only parts of Fantasyland, Tomorrowland, and some of the other "lands"—plus all those big "Mickeys" and "Minnies" and "Donalds" and "Cinderellas" that walk right up to you and shake your hand. I'd love to go back again.

SUPERBOWL: I'm a football fan and I like to go to the Jets games in New York with my orthopedic surgeon Dr. Nicholas (who is also orthopedist for the Jets) and his wife, Kiki. I'd never been to a Super-

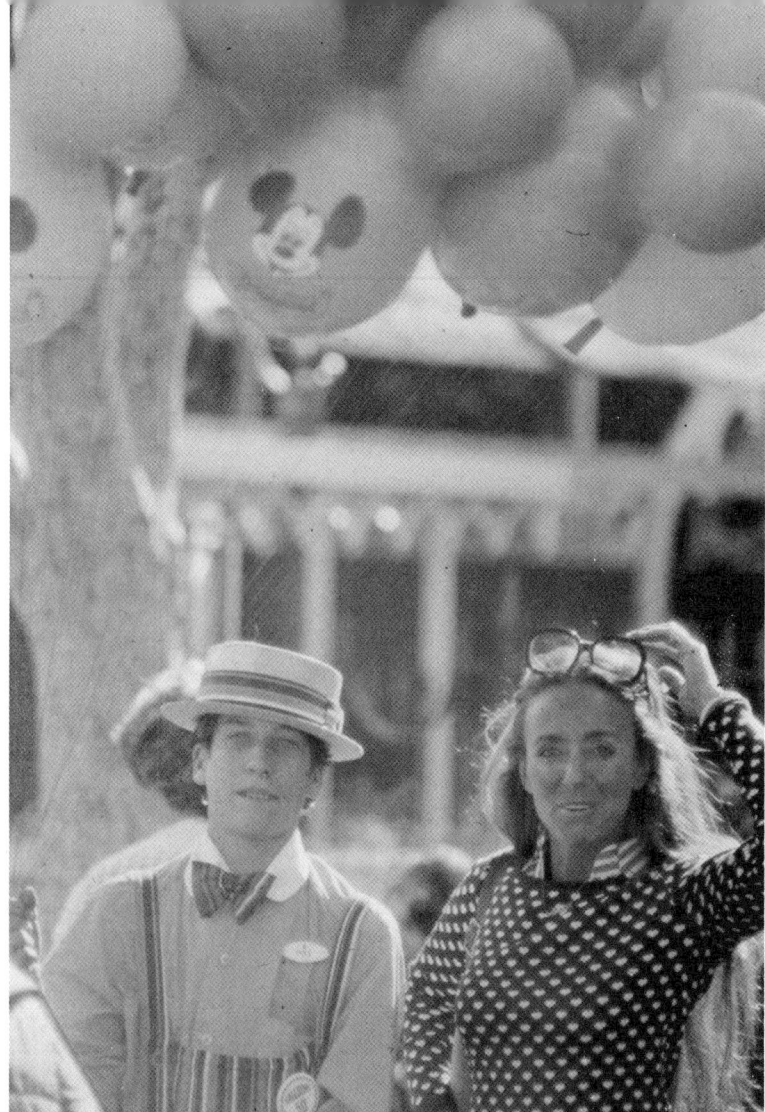

You don't have to be under twelve years old to love Disneyland. (PHOTO: LEE GUBER)

bowl until 1976. It was a one-of-a-kind experience in more ways than one. Joan and Alan Cohen invited me and we sat on the shady side of the stadium—purposely, to avoid sitting in the hot sun. But the temperature went down to 25 or 30 that day. For that kind of weather you need sweaters and a fur coat. I sat there shivering, teeth chattering through the whole game. I was so cold, I can't remember who won.

MONTREAL: An utterly charming, utterly European city, just forty-five minutes from New York by plane. With its little bistros, the sound of

French spoken everywhere, at times it was like being in Paris. I went there for the Olympics during the summer of 1976. Another first for me, another one-of-a-kind experience.

The athletes, all of them, were dazzling. The new Olympic stadium is one of the best designed I've ever seen. I couldn't help but be struck by the courtesy of the crowds. At the end of each day, people filed out slowly, almost reluctantly. Perhaps it was difficult for them to tear themselves away from the spectacle. I know that's how it was for me.

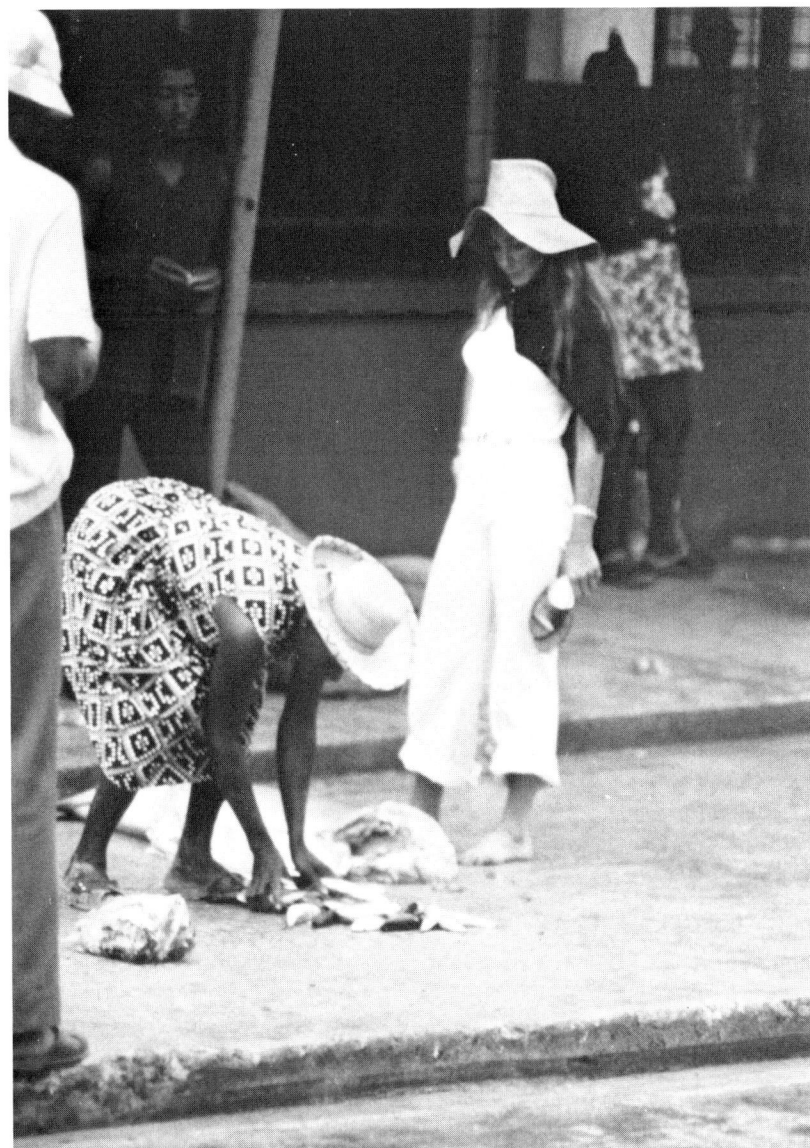

Buying flying fish (a great delicacy) in Barbados. (PHOTO: LEE GUBER)

BARBADOS: It's a heavenly place for the beach person, with its miles and miles of smooth white sand and tepid clear blue water. It's a place to relax, get a tan, eat (and get fat, too, if you don't watch out). When I think of Barbados, I think of beach and food, especially flying fish.

They tell me that the weather is consistently sunny and warm in Barbados, and I'm sure that it's true—for most of the time. But once when I was there it rained and rained for days and the streets became miniature canals.

Last time, the time it rained, I was the guest of former Mayor and Mrs. Robert Wagner who each year rent a house near the town of Spitesville. It is a tribute and a credit to the Wagners that in spite of the rain we had a splendid time. All of us—the Wagners, their son Bob, Jr., Donna Shalala, Lee Guber, and I—spent long, lazy mornings gathering shells and green beach glass—the kind that is smoothed and polished by years of being dashed by waves against the shore. At the beach, we often ran into the Wagners' next-door neighbor Claudette Colbert—still marvelous-looking with those high, high cheekbones. At night, I was thrilled to meet author Lillian Hellman.

(Back at home, I gave two of the largest pieces of green glass we'd collected to jeweler Julius Cohen, who is a very fine jeweler. He polished the glass and cut one piece into a heart shape, the other into a number "1." Then he outlined each in gold and hung them on delicate gold chains. The resulting pendants have some of the cool green beauty of emeralds. I gave the pendant with the heart-shaped glass to Phyllis Wagner, who collects hearts. The number "1" I gave to Donna.)

In Barbados, the Sandy Lane Hotel is a wonderful place to stay. Not too far away is a tiny museum with a collection of exquisite little shell-covered wooden boxes made long ago by sailors for their wives and sweethearts.

JONES BEACH: New Yorkers don't have to go to Rio to find a good beach. We've got one of the best right here (well, not exactly smack in Manhattan, but out on Long Island, an hour away by car). I'm talking about Jones Beach.

I think many Americans don't realize how great are the beaches in this country. It's hard to find a good beach in Europe. The famous

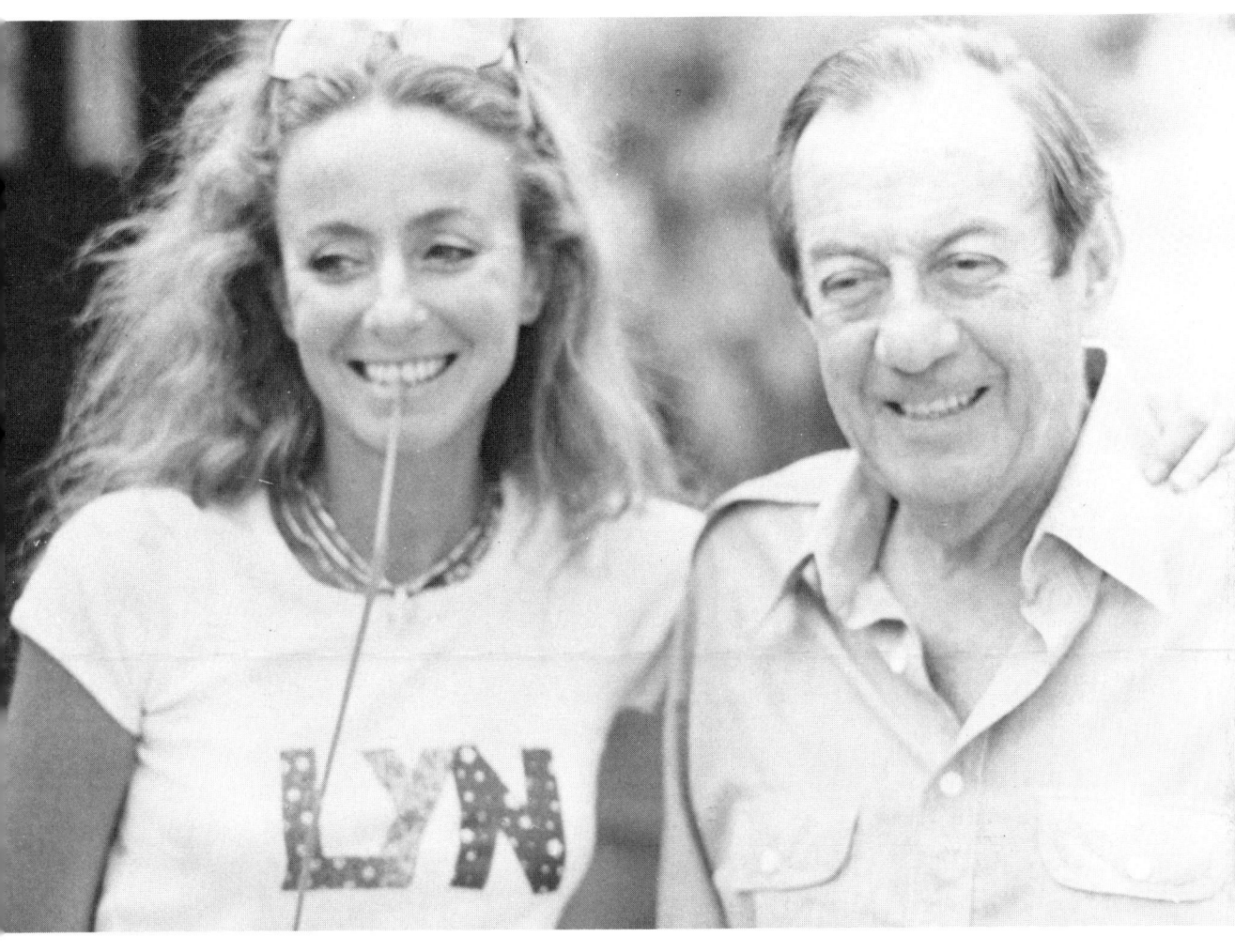

In Barbados with former New York City Mayor Robert F. Wagner . . .

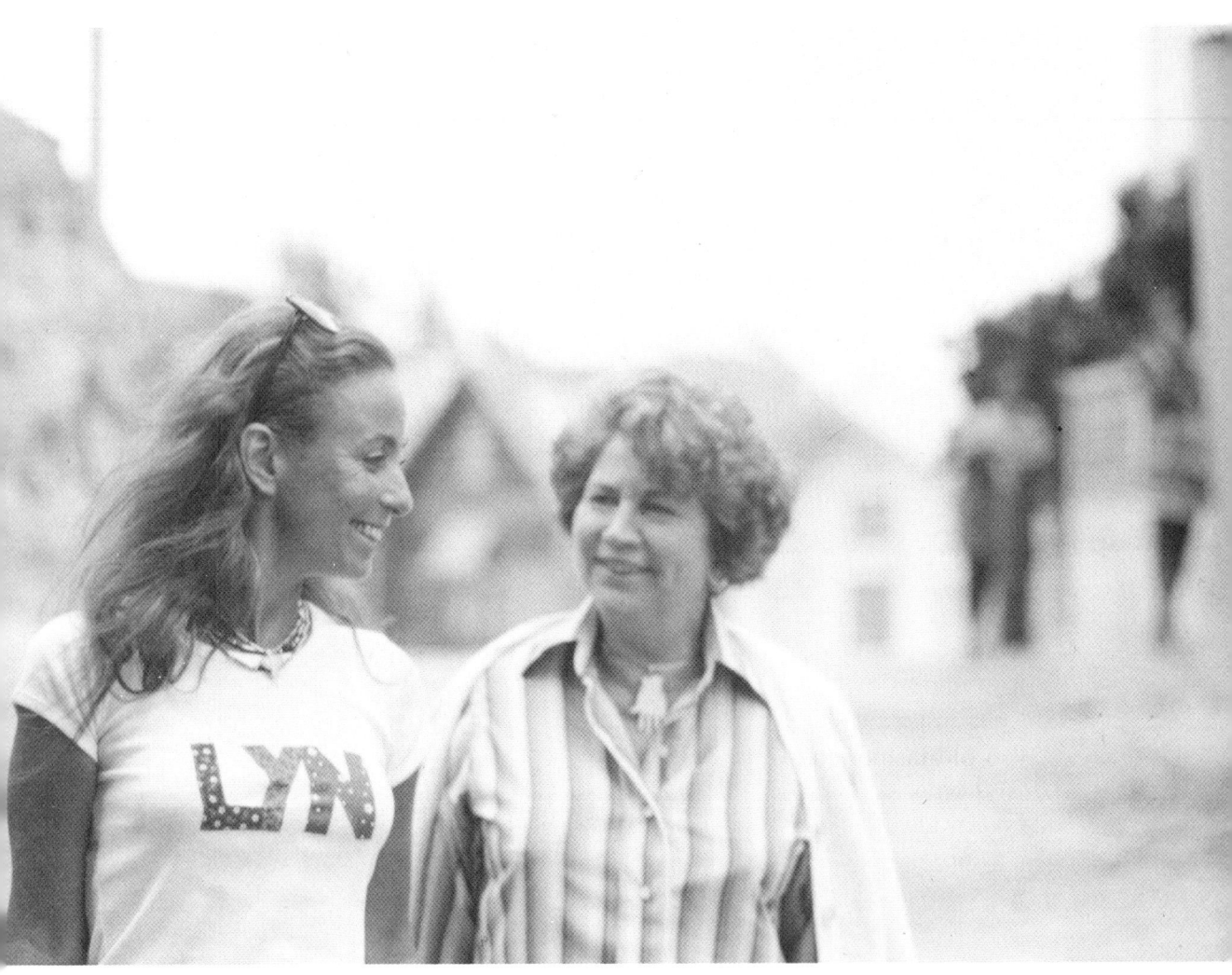
and Phyllis Wagner (PHOTO: LEE GUBER)

beach at Nice is just a tiny strip of rocks. At Monte Carlo they think they have a beach, but it's just rocks. They say Copacabana Beach in Rio is beautiful but I wouldn't know. When I went there it was so packed with bodies I never saw the sand. (It was December then, summer in Brazil, and 120 humid degrees.) Jones Beach is something else again. Not much glamor, but great sand, great water.

My enthusiasm for Jones Beach goes back to one summer when the boys were away at camp and Susan (who was too young to go with them) and I spent the summer in town. One day we went out in search of a beach and found a great white powdery stretch of it at Jones (which is really a series of beaches, each with its own parking lot and other facilities). We spent practically every sunny day there, sitting in the sun, playing in the sand.

The way I go on about beaches, you'd think I was an ace swimmer. The truth is I don't swim a stroke. As a child I went away to camp ten years in a row. At the end of each year they got me to float, but by the next year I had to start all over again from the beginning. I was the only thirteen-year-old camper with a five-year-old buddy.

MARRIAGE: In many ways I'm not the woman of today. I believe that the most important jobs for a woman are caring for her husband and children, and that these at certain stages in life are full-time jobs. I am also old-fashioned in that I believe in marriage. I believe that a man and woman can be happy in marriage. I believe there can be love and fidelity and trust between them. It takes work and concentration, but it is possible.